THREE PATIENTS

International Perspective on
Intensive Care at the
End of Life

THREE PATIENTS

International Perspective on Intensive Care at the End of Life

Edited by

David Crippen, MD
Jack K. Kilcullen, MD, JD, MPH
David F. Kelly, PhD

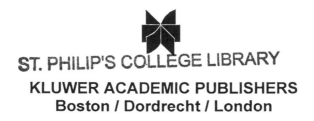

KLUWER ACADEMIC PUBLISHERS
Boston / Dordrecht / London

Distributors for North, Central and South America:
Kluwer Academic Publishers
101 Philip Drive
Assinippi Park
Norwell, Massachusetts 02061 USA
Telephone (781) 871-6600
Fax (781) 681-9045
E-Mail <kluwer@wkap.com>

Distributors for all other countries:
Kluwer Academic Publishers Group
Post Office Box 322
3300 AH Dordrecht, THE NETHERLANDS
Telephone 31-786-576-000
Fax 31-786-576-254
E-Mail <services@wkap.nl>

 Electronic Services <http://www.wkap.nl>

Library of Congress Cataloging-in-Publication Data

Three patients : international perspective on intensive care at the end of life / edited by
David Crippen, Jack K. Kilcullen, David F. Kelly.
    p. ; cm.
  Includes bibliographical references and index.
  ISBN 0-7923-7671-4 (hardback : alk. paper)
   1. Euthanasia--Cross-cultural studies. 2. Right to die--Cross-cultural studies. 3. Critical
care medicine--Cross-cultural studies. 4. Medical ethics--Cross-cultural studies. I.
Crippen, David, 1943- II. Kilcullen, Jack K. III. Kelly, David F.
  [DNLM: 1. Euthanasia, Passive--Case Report. 2. Cross-Cultural Comparison--Case
Report. 3. Ethics, Clinical--Case Report. 4. Intensive Care--utilization--Case Report. 5.
Right to Die--Case Report. W 50 T531 2002]
R726 .T49 2002
174'.24--dc21

                                                  2002016051

Printed on acid-free paper.
Printed in the United States of America

The Publisher offers discounts on this book for course use and bulk purchases.
For further information, send email to melissa.ramondetta@wkap.com.

Contents

Introduction

Multinational Perspective
on Treatment of the Three Patients

Summaries of Medical Comments

Patient A

Patient B

Patient C

General Multidisciplinary Survey

Comments From Paramedical Providers

Contributors

Anna Batchelor, MB, ChB
Consultant, Department of Anaesthesia and Intensive Care Medicine, Royal Victoria Infirmary, Newcastle, United Kingdom

Rolando Berger, MD
Professor, Division of Pulmonary Medicine, University of Kentucky Medical Center, Lexington, Kentucky

Richard Burrows, MB, BCh
Intensivist, Intensive Care Unit, Addington Hospital, Durban, South Africa

Don Chalfin, MD
Director, Division of Research; Attending Intensivist, Department of Emergency Medicine, Maimonides Medical Center, Brooklyn, New York

David Crippen, MD
Associate Director, Departments of Emergency and Critical Care Medicine, St. Francis Medical Center, Pittsburgh, Pennsylvania

Ivor S. Douglas, MD
Assistant Professor, Pulmonary, Allergy and Critical Care Medicine, New York Presbyterian Hospital, Columbia University College of Physicians & Surgeons, New York, New York

Malcolm Fisher, MD
Medical Director, Intensive Care Unit, Royal North Shore Hospital, St. Leonards, New South Wales, Australia

Gabriele Ford, CCRN
Staff Nurse, Sacred Heart Medical Center, Eugene, Oregon

Bruce Gipe, MD
Medical Director, Primary Critical Care Medical Group, North Hollywood, California

John W. Hoyt, MD
Clinical Professor, Department of Anesthesiology and Critical Care
Medicine, University of Pittsburgh Medical School; Chairman, Department
of Critical Care Medicine, St. Francis Medical Center, Pittsburgh,
Pennsylvania

Leslie Beckhart Jenal, JD
Chaplain, UCLA Medical Center, Los Angeles, California

Farhad Kapadia, MD
Consultant Physician and Intensivist, Intensive Care Units, Hinduja
Hospital, Mahim, Bombay, India

Michael Karakozov, MD
Staff Intensivist, Intensive Care Unit, Karelian Republican Clinic,
Petrozavodsk, Karelia, Russia

David F. Kelly, PhD
Director, Health Care Ethics Center, Duquesne University, Pittsburgh,
Pennsylvania

Jack K. Kilcullen, MD, JD, MPH
Fellow, Division of Critical Care Medicine, Albert Einstein College of
Medicine, Montefiore Medical Center, Bronx, New York

Mitchell Levy, MD
Associate Director, Medical Intensive Care Unit, Brown University Medical
Center, Providence, Rhode Island

Ted S. Rogovein, MD
Director, Intensive Care Unit, St. Joseph's Health Centre, Toronto, Ontario,
Canada

Aviel Roy-Shapira, MD
Surgeon and Intensivist, Departments of Surgery and Critical Care, Soroka
University Hospital; Ben-Gurion University Medical School, Beersheba,
Israel

Peter Safar, MD
Professor and Director, International Resuscitation Research Center,
Pittsburgh, Pennsylvania

Stephen Streat, MD
Intensivist, Department of Critical Care Medicine, Auckland Hospital, Auckland, New Zealand

Ian K.S. Tan, MBBS
Director, Intensive Care Unit, Pamela Youde Nethersole Eastern Hospital; Adjunct Associate Professor, Chinese University of Hong Kong, Chai Wan, Hong Kong SAR, People's Republic of China

Hans van der Spoel, MD
Intensivist, Department of Intensive Care, Onze Lieve Vrouwe Gasthuis, Amsterdam, the Netherlands

Jean-Louis Vincent, MD
Head, Department of Intensive Care, Erasme University Hospital, Free University of Brussels, Brussels, Belgium

David H. Walker, MA, RRT, RCP
Chief Technology Officer, Valley Children's Hospital, Fresno, California

Foreword

Peter Safar, MD

This book uses a novel approach, including discussion of three cases by
critical care physicians from around the world, to address some of the
ethical dilemmas stemming from modern medical technology and the
lifesaving potentials of modern critical care medicine. Patient A, the first of
the three patients, deserves all-out intensive care throughout. Patient B
illustrates the need for the intensivist to recognize when the fight for
meaningful survival is lost. Patient C illustrates futility from the start.
Thoughtful reading of this text by health care professionals and laypersons
may help reduce inappropriate use of critical care resources. The differences
in approaches that various physicians propose for the three patients
described in this book help to clarify confusing ethical issues. Ideally,
physicians themselves should be ethicists and should be equipped to guide
lawyers.

Critical care (also called intensive care) is medical care, preferably
multidisciplinary, for critically ill or injured patients, plus coordinated
intensive nursing care that involves assistance by members of other
professions as well. The goal has always been to achieve long-term survival
without brain damage.[1] Intensive care must be administered according to
pathophysiologic derangements and therapeutic potentials, with caretakers
constantly present. Critical care differs from standard medical practice, in
which physicians make rounds (or patients visit doctors' offices), prescribe,
and leave. Ideally, critical care encompasses more than the interventions that
take place in the hospital intensive care unit (ICU). Critical care is
cardiopulmonary cerebral resuscitation[2] and a progression of basic,
advanced, and prolonged life support. Critical care includes prevention
(through monitoring and life support) and reversal (through emergency
resuscitation) of acute terminal states (e.g., asphyxiation, shock, or multiple
organ failure), as well as prevention of sudden death (e.g., from cardiac
arrest). The ultimate goal of critical care is to preserve the viability of vital
organs long enough to give nature and curative treatments a chance to
correct the underlying disorder, resulting in survival with mentation.

One problem now facing intensivists is that application of available and effective resuscitation and life-support methods is still suboptimal, often too little too late. For example, in the case of sudden coma or shock, an immediate emergency resuscitation attempt can be life saving and can reduce the need for expensive, long-term intensive care. A second problem is that expensive technologies are often applied inappropriately in ICUs, with the use of such technologies being continued when there is no longer any chance of survival without brain damage. The reasons for this are many, including physician pride (or lack of knowledge), unreasonable demands by the family (or, less often, by the patient), reimbursement objectives of hospital administration, interests of consultants, and fear of lawsuits.

The history of critical care medicine can teach important lessons concerning the ethics regarding these challenges.[1-6] Until the Renaissance, most human societies considered acute dying to be the will of God. This acceptance of acute, unexpected death appeared to be in conflict with Judeo-Christian views of the sanctity of human life and the duty to help others survive. Since the Renaissance, there has been a will to achieve resuscitation, although effective methods were elusive until the 1950s. The introduction in the late 1800s of general anesthesia—which can cause airway obstruction, cessation of breathing, and pulselessness—and the improvement of trauma care during World War II prompted searches for increasingly more effective methods of resuscitation. In the 1950s, these efforts culminated in the ability to reverse dying processes, with this reversal often commencing outside the hospital. At the same time that external cardiopulmonary resuscitation was introduced,[3] patients paralyzed by poliomyelitis[4] or comatose from intoxications[5] began receiving prolonged mechanical artificial ventilation. Since 1958, patients with failure of any vital organ have received multidisciplinary, physician-guided intensive-care life support.[6] Religious leaders have agreed with anesthesiologists and intensivists since the 1950s that it is ethical to discontinue artificial ventilation in the presence of brain death and to discontinue "extraordinary measures" in the absence of any chance of conscious survival. Beyond those seemingly clear-cut decisions, many intensivists in the early years used a mix of paternalism and common sense to avoid administering senseless, protracted, expensive intensive care.

Ethical dilemmas created by the lifesaving potentials of modern critical care medicine have multiplied since the 1950s, as a result of increasingly potent life-support measures—including treatment with novel drugs, more effective prolonged support of circulation (such as with an artificial heart), and organ transplantation—and in response to irrational or uninformed demands made by families of unconscious (incompetent) patients or by conscious (competent) patients themselves for treatments not medically indicated and lacking in benefit.

Several ethical principles have evolved that could reduce the inappropriate use of critical care[7-10]: 1) Determining the appropriate level of care (all-out resuscitation and life support, general medical care, general nursing care only, or terminal care) is a medical decision that the physician must make in discussion with the patient or proxy.[8] 2) The physician does not have to authorize life support that he or she considers futile.[9] 3) The intensivist should do his or her best for the patient—using available resources, which are always finite. 4) Situations of emergency resuscitation usually allow no time for contemplation and consultation to determine a patient's resuscitability; however, after an initial all-out emergency resuscitation attempt and stabilization of spontaneous circulation, the salvageability and appropriate level of care should be determined before initiating protracted, potentially expensive, prolonged life support. After cardiac arrest and resuscitation, the decision to let a patient die can often be made clinically by as early as 3–7 days. 5) In cases of long-term life support for persistent vegetative state (permanent coma without brain death), all support, including artificial feeding, hydration, and antibiotic therapy, should be withheld to allow the patient to die in dignity.[9] 6) Critical care resources should be used for those who can benefit most, with the focus being on recovery of mentation. 7) All-out intensive care, if considered futile, is contraindicated not only because it is wasteful but also because it is undignified and a potential source of torture for patient, family, friends, and caregivers. 8) With regard to limiting life support, the informed patient's autonomy should be respected. 9) When the decision to let a patient die is supported by the patient, family, intensivist, and primary physician, terminal care should be adjusted moment to moment and must not only be compassionate but also respect the dignity of patient, family, friends, and caregivers. This is possible not only in the hospice setting but also in the ICU. 10) The greatest dilemmas are posed by the increasing number of patients whose personalities are destroyed by Alzheimer's disease and severe dementia in very old age.[10] These patients most often are not appropriate candidates for ICU admission.

In a humane, ethical society, *basic* health care must be provided irrespective of the individual's ability to pay. The basics provided by a national health care system (in the United States, perhaps a Medicare for all) must include emergency resuscitation and long-term intensive care for critically ill or injured patients when there is a reasonable chance of conscious survival. Beyond the basics, national insurance can cover only care that is available regionally; some rationing is unavoidable. The basics must be defined by wise physicians. Limiting services in order to benefit society and returning excess revenues into not-for-profit health care systems are ethical. Limiting needed medical services in order to increase corporate profits is not. In the United States, patients often demand (and perhaps receive) whatever is available, irrespective of cost; elsewhere, decisions regarding level and cost of care are often not left entirely to the patient.

How to handle a lack of agreement on the appropriate level of care is a focus of discussions in this book. *Patient autonomy* refers to the individual's right to refuse any recommended treatment. Patient autonomy does not include the right to receive therapy that is not medically indicated. In my work as an intensivist, I have never encountered a rational person who wanted an emergency resuscitation attempt not to be made if there was a chance to survive with good brain function (depressed patients and patients in the terminal state of an incurable disease or in severe pain excepted), nor have I encountered a patient who wanted to have long-term life support continued when there was no chance to survive without brain damage. Living wills cannot anticipate the specific conditions at the end of life. Therefore, it is advisable to appoint as proxies a friend or relative plus a trusted physician.

Principle 5, described earlier and relating to prognostication and decision making in the case of coma, calls both for continued dialogue on ethics and for basic pathophysiologic research. We should move beyond reliance on epidemiologic correlation statistics that ignore the individual.

When faced with the possibility of irreversible brain damage, we still cannot prognosticate with 100% accuracy when life support will not bring about recovery. Survival is a goal in cases of cerebral performance category (CPC) 1 (normal function) or 2 (mild to moderate disability but self-sustaining). Rather than merely estimate using epidemiologic statistics, we must learn to prognosticate permanent CPC 3 (severe disability but conscious) or permanent CPC 4 (coma or vegetative state) using patho-physiologic measurements. In the meantime, we must use epidemiologic statistics, experience, and judgment—that is, all of the art of medicine. If critical care medicine is practiced with scientific knowledge, reason, and compassion, it will indeed be a positive force in the evolution of humanism.

References

[1]Grenvik A, Ayres SM, Holbrook PR, et al (eds): Textbook of Critical Care Medicine. 4th ed. Philadelphia, PA: WB Saunders, 2000.

[2]Safar P, Bircher NG: Cardiopulmonary Cerebral Resuscitation: An Introduction to Resuscitation Medicine. 3rd ed. London: WB Saunders, 1988.

[3]Safar P: On the history of modern resuscitation. Crit Care Med 1996;24:S3–11.

[4]Ibsen B: The anaesthetist's viewpoint on treatment of respiratory complications in poliomyelitis during the epidemic in Copenhagen, 1952. Proc R Soc Med 1954;47:72–4.

[5]Nilsson E: On treatment of barbiturate poisoning. A modified clinical aspect. Acta Med Scand 1951;253 (suppl):1.

[6]Safar P, DeKornfeld TJ, Pearson JW, et al: Intensive care unit. Anaesthesia 1961;16:275–84.

[7]Safar P: The physician's responsibility towards hopelessly critically ill patients. Ethical dilemmas in resuscitation medicine. Acta Anaesthesiol Scand 1991;35 (suppl 96):147–9.

[8]Grenvik A, Powner DJ, Snyder JV, et al: Cessation of therapy in terminal illness and brain death. Crit Care Med 1978;6:284–91.

[9]President's Commission for the Study of Ethical Problems in Medicine and Biomedical and Behavioral Research: Deciding to Forego Life-Sustaining Treatment: A Report on the Ethical, Medical and Legal Issues in Treatment Decisions. Washington, DC: U.S. Government Printing Office, 1983, p 232.

[10]Wanzer SH, Adelstein SJ, Cranford RE, et al: The physician's responsibility toward hopelessly ill patients. N Engl J Med 1984;310:955–9.

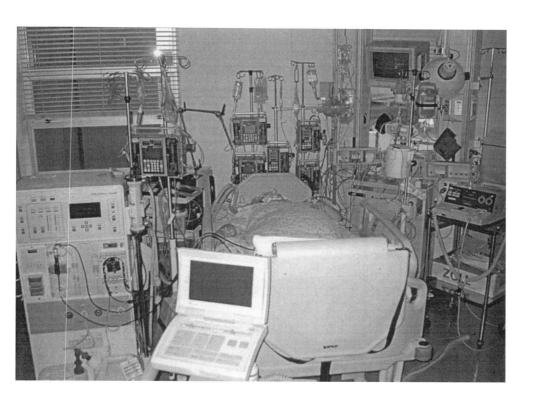

Introduction

Overview

Jack K. Kilcullen, MD, JD, MPH

The intensive care unit (ICU) is a world apart. To families, it is feared foreign territory, where even entry to see a loved one is tightly regulated. That loved one is often unconscious, misshaped by fluids, and immobilized by countless tubes. To general physicians caring for patients just beyond its doors, the ICU is a corridor filled with an intimidating battery of new technology that seemingly renders inadequate the doctor's simple touch. To patients, the ICU is often a world of dark and drifting shadows and sounds, punctuated by blinding jabs of pain.

At the heart of the ICU lies a mission no less confounding: do everything. Ever more sensitive monitors, ventilators equipped with more powerful microprocessors, and therapies that replicate the body's most sophisticated enzymes are brought to the bedside of the hospital's sickest patients in the hope of new promise.

Yet ironies blossom with no less flourish than a resistant micro-organism. Despite all the research poured into intensive care, it has been estimated that less than 25% of standard practice is based on Class I evidence—findings of double-blind, randomized controlled studies (V. Kvetan, oral communication, May 2001). Much else is extrapolated from animal data, small population studies, and accepted general practice. Moreover, methodologies, often invasive and costly, have been allowed to become standard practice well before there were data to support them. For example, thousands of pulmonary artery catheters were inserted into patients who entered the ICU, before research began to suggest that their widespread use was associated with poorer outcomes.[1] Now they are far more selectively employed.

Furthermore, the bane of critical care—severe sepsis—remains a relentless foe.[2] Despite researchers' vast understanding of the cellular events, standard therapy has changed little in decades, still centering around fluid resuscitation, antibiotics, and vasopressors.[3]

As a result, even when doctors "do everything," patients die. Although ICU protocols have cut deeply into mortality rates for numerous conditions, there will always be people who come to the hospital too sick to save. Intracranial hemorrhage, massive myocardial infarction, and sudden gastro-intestinal bleeding can snatch a life as the wind snatches a leaf.

The sharpest irony, though, occurs when intensive care can only continue life without saving the patient. When the brain has been starved for oxygen long enough to leave lifeless the circuitry that gives shape to personality and purpose, its primitive centers regulating the body may persist. The best intensive care may leave the patient able to breathe and digest but do precious little else. As a result, the body is newly vulnerable to infections and decay without the careful maintenance provided by others. Continuing intensive care for such a patient can only prolong a false sense of what treatment can accomplish.

Many patients and their families know the truth they face. Through the hospice movement or through cultural traditions that long preceded modern medicine, many facing death may do so at home with those they love. Physicians have slowly begun to respond to this desire for death with dignity, developing specialized treatments to ease suffering, treatments referred to collectively as palliative care.

The difficulty is when there is no shared understanding between physicians and patients and their families. Providing patients with care that will never return to them any scrap of their former lives tears at the ethical standards of physicians not to give treatment they consider futile. Yet when some doctors and hospitals have withdrawn care, they have been sued by surviving family members.[4]

But can and should physicians "do everything" on the basis of only a patient's real or perceived wish? In the United States, health care costs have made up an increasing share of the gross domestic product. After that percentage increased from 10% to 14% between 1984 and the early 1990s, managed care and federal cutbacks held spending down until the early part of this century, when it took off once more; it is estimated that by 2010, health care expenditures will make up 16% of the country's gross domestic product.[5] Despite the billions spent, the World Health Organization ranked the United States 15th in attainment of health indicators and a shocking 37th in efficiency, behind not just the countries of western Europe but also Chile and Colombia.[6] Perhaps the greatest flaw in the United States is the inequity in access to health care: 41 million Americans do not have health insurance, a situation that creates a chasm between haves and have-nots.

As the population ages, the demand for intensive care is expected to increase dramatically, whereas the supply of physicians trained in critical care medicine will lag.[7] Absent an increase in staffing and beds, competition for an ICU bed will stiffen dramatically over the next three decades. For those intensivists who control access to their ICUs, the ethical demands are unique; nowhere else in the health care system, outside the field of organ transplantation, are physicians called on to choose patients for treatment from among desperately ill people. Hospital committees in charge of allocating donated organs apply clear protocols and have painstaking discussions before deciding eligibility. By contrast, the ICU physician must decide whom to admit, transfer, or reject, often alone, often at night, and often in response to a shifting demand for beds. Ethical guidelines may be so cautiously worded that they offer no practical help.

What complicates this already impossible situation is that the patient and family often have no understanding of what is taking place. Treatment is the patient's right if he or she has insurance to pay for it. Even when the patient's insurance or lack thereof restricts him or her to public facilities, the patient still expects a bed in the ICU; the concept of competing for the bed itself is not at all apparent.

For ICU physicians, these ethical tangles that are so foreign even to other physicians are a daily part of a frustrating world, especially when these intensivists have limited control over access to the ICU. They see the patients who cannot get in because a bed is taken by someone who cannot be treated, yet cannot be moved.

The debate over medically futile treatment is not new. It has skated across numerous journals over the past 20 years.[8] On one side of the debate are those who would grant physicians authority in determining how long effective treatment should continue. On the other side are those who maintain that such decisions are not scientific but are ultimately subjective and that a respect for patient autonomy should determine the extent of care.

In this book, the debate is planted squarely in the ICU, where the urgency to resolve it mounts yearly. First Dr. Kelly presents an introduction to the arguments over medically futile treatment in the United States. Then three fictitious patients arrive in turn at the ICU, each critically ill but with a different degree of promise. A panel of experienced critical care physicians from around the world offer their assessments and propose management based on resources they routinely have. Then they describe what they would do with unlimited resources. Their insights are provocative in part because most of these physicians work in national health care systems with universal access to finite resources. In nations with tight budgets, maximizing care means careful consideration of the patient most likely to benefit. To physicians from those countries, the concept of patient autonomy and moving care away from patients with a greater chance of survival is as foreign as health care rationing is to the average American patient.

Following the descriptions of medical management of each case is a separate analysis, contrasting the issues raised by the international contributors. Afterward, Dr. Crippen discusses the moral issues of intensive care management and how the distortions in United States health care financing impede effective use of ICU beds. Then Dr. Kelly lays the historical foundation of the overarching ethical issues and the resultant clash of perspective between patient and physician. I subsequently review existing legal precedents and describe how recent federal legislation actually aggravates the conflict. A nursing perspective on end-of-life issues is provided by Ms. Ford, the view of a respiratory therapist by Mr. Walker, and that of a hospital chaplain by Ms. Jenal. Dr. Crippen concludes the book with a view toward the future and a discussion of the need to take up the challenge before the crisis stage arrives.

Most importantly, through this collective enterprise, we seek to open wide the doors into the ICU so that both the public and the policy makers can see the daily reality of caring for critically ill people. We wish to show how these daily decisions affect what society has to offer patients in years soon to come.

References

[1]Connors AF Jr, Speroff T, Dawson NV, et al: The effectiveness of right heart catheterization in the initial care of critically ill patients. SUPPORT Investigators. JAMA 1996;276:889–97.

[2]Brun-Buisson C, Doyon F, Carlet J, et al: Incidence, risk factors, and outcome of severe sepsis and septic shock in adults. A multicenter prospective study in intensive care units. French ICU Group for Severe Sepsis. JAMA 1995;274:968–74.

[3]Practice parameters for hemodynamic support of sepsis in adult patients in sepsis. Task Force of the American College of Critical Care Medicine, Society of Critical Care Medicine. Crit Care Med 1999;27:639–60.

[4]*Causey v St. Francis Med. Ctr.,* 719 So2d 1072 (1998) La App LEXIS 2477 (La App 2d Cir [1998]).

[5]Heffler S, Levit K, Smith S, et al: Health spending growth up in 1999; faster growth expected in the future. Health Aff (Millwood) 2001;20:193–203.

[6]The World Health Report 2000. Health Systems: Improving Performance. Geneva: World Health Organization, 2000.

[7]Angus DC, Kelley MA, Schmitz RJ, et al: Caring for the critically ill patient. Current and projected workforce requirements for care of the critically ill and patients with pulmonary disease: can we meet the requirements of an aging population? JAMA 2000;284:2762–70.

[8]Helft PR, Siegler M, Lantos J: The rise and fall of the futility movement. N Engl J Med 2000;343:293–6.

Medical Futility
in American Health Care

David F. Kelly, PhD

When I began consulting at a major tertiary medical center in September 1989 during a sabbatical year, I had a number of anticipations about what I would find, some explicit and many implicit. One of these anticipations was that in most instances of conflict about forgoing treatment between health care providers and patients or patient surrogates, providers would insist on initiating or continuing aggressive therapy, and patients—or, more often, patients' families—would ask to have useless or burdensome treatment withheld or discontinued. The medical ethical literature I had read suggested that in cases of conflict, the physicians' medical approach would be set against the more humane moral sense of patients and families. I anticipated that physicians, and possibly other health care providers, would see disease and death as the main enemies and would try to hold them off at all costs. It would be the families who would ask that their loved ones be allowed to die with dignity, without disproportionate use of medication and technology.

What I found was more often the opposite. Though such conflicts did and sometimes still do arise, there had been a major shift in the type of conflictive case. The most contentious cases were usually those in which the family insisted on aggressive treatments and the physicians wanted to stop treatment. Often the physicians argued that treatments were futile. The present debate about the meaning of and the criteria for medical futility arose as a result of such conflicts.

The American Consensus on Forgoing Treatment

There are three pillars of the present American consensus on forgoing treatment. The first pillar is the general agreement by most Americans that not all medical treatment that prolongs biological life is of human benefit to the patient. Not all agree, but most do. This pillar relies historically on a distinction, long applied in Roman Catholic medical ethics, between ordinary and extraordinary means of treatment. Persons are obliged to use ordinary (or reasonable or proportionate) means to preserve or prolong their lives, but not extraordinary (or unreasonable or disproportionate) means. In the context of medical futility, it is particularly important to note that this distinction is a moral one and not a medical one. Thus, what might be a reasonable or ordinary treatment for a person who has a decent chance of recovery might well be unreasonable or extraordinary for a person whose chance of recovery is less. It is not the technical or medical characteristic of the treatment itself, nor even its immediate medical effect, that determines whether it is ordinary and hence morally mandatory, or extraordinary and hence morally optional. An otherwise healthy person who develops pneumonia is said by the received Catholic tradition to be obliged to take antibiotics, but a person with terminal cancer who develops pneumonia need not. The same medical treatment with the same immediate medical effect—cure of pneumonia—is morally ordinary in one case and morally extraordinary in another.

Though there is some debate about whether to use the terms *ordinary* and *extraordinary,* the general American consensus is in accordance with the Catholic position that it is not necessary to do everything possible to preserve life. The obligation to use ordinary means rests with the person himself or herself. American law goes further than this, of course, and gives patients the legal right to refuse even beneficial treatments.

The second pillar is the distinction between killing (euthanasia) and allowing to die. Legally, killing a patient is criminal, and the Catholic tradition, which again has been influential in bringing Americans to this agreement, has held that killing an innocent person, as for example in euthanasia, is always morally wrong. Though many now disagree and are working toward legalization of euthanasia and physician-assisted suicide, thus far the United States has generally agreed that it is always wrong to kill a dying patient and sometimes right to allow a dying patient to die.

Thus, when it is appropriate to withhold treatment, the withholding may be followed by the patient's death. But it is the disease that kills the patient. Withholding in this context is allowing to die, not killing. The same is true of withdrawing treatment. The two are morally equivalent, other things being equal. Finally, sedation for pain may hasten death—as in cases in which sedation contributes to respiratory insufficiency—but it is not considered killing when the intention is to reduce pain and when no more medication is given than is needed for the pain. It is always possible and it is ethically right and legally right, provided the patient or family agrees, to eliminate physical pain in the patient facing imminent death. Reasons sometimes used in claiming that there are exceptions, such as fear of addiction or fear of respiratory depression, are not justification for refusing pain relief for a patient about to die. American hospitals are very good at administering technologically advanced aggressive therapies but often very bad at pain management.

Thus, withholding or withdrawing treatment and sedation for pain are not the same as active euthanasia. They are by no means always right, but they may be, and often are. The *Cruzan* decision (June 1990)[1] and the assisted-suicide decisions (June 1997) of the United States Supreme Court made that very clear. Killing the patient by direct euthanasia, on the other hand, is illegal in all states, and assisted suicide is explicitly illegal in many states, implicitly illegal in many more, and legal only in Oregon.

The third pillar is the American legal concept of privacy and autonomy and of liberty to refuse treatment. It is clear in American law that patients capable of deciding may forgo just about any treatment.[2] Patients not capable of deciding may have this decision made by surrogates. When a surrogate makes the decision, that decision must be in the patient's best interests or the decision that the patient would have made if he or she were able (substituted judgment based on known wishes of the patient). The best interests standard translates in some sense into the difference between reasonable and unreasonable or ordinary and extraordinary treatment. Whereas a patient himself or herself may legally forgo reasonable or morally mandatory treatment, a surrogate may decide that a patient is to forgo only unreasonable or clearly extraordinary means of preserving life.

Medical Futility

Importance of the Issue

There are two major areas of controversy concerning the American consensus on forgoing treatment. One is legalization of physician-assisted suicide and euthanasia. In the United States, such legalization has thus far occurred only in Oregon. It undermines the second pillar I discussed. The other area of controversy, the topic here, concerns medical futility and consists of the proposal to allow physicians, on the basis of their medical knowledge, to reject certain treatments desired by patients or surrogates. This proposal thus argues for changes in the third pillar underlying the consensus, the procedural or legal pillar supporting the right of the patient or surrogate to decide about treatment options. Attempts have recently been made to develop criteria for determining medical futility that would expand the applicability of the concept.

I began this discussion with one indication of the importance of this topic: the shift in the kind of conflict case from the older typical case in which the physician insists on aggressive treatment against the family's wishes, to the newer case in which the patient or family insists on treatment against the advice of the health care team. The large number of articles dealing with the topic indicates that the shift is a general phenomenon. Physicians and ethicists are increasingly interested in what to do when physicians want to stop treatment and families want to continue. My conversations with health care providers at various hospitals have led me to believe that this shift has occurred more in urban hospitals than in rural ones. That is, physicians in rural hospitals are apt to continue insisting on aggressive treatment for terminally ill patients despite family wishes, whereas in urban hospitals, families are more apt to insist on such treatment, and physicians tend to want to discontinue aggressive treatment. It is probable that changes like this one occur first in urban teaching centers and eventually in rural institutions.

Why the shift? I believe there are three reasons. First, American health care providers have become more aware of the importance of patient autonomy. There is a greater emphasis on informed consent and other issues of patients' rights. Certain decisions about treatment are made by the patient or the patient's surrogate. These decisions are not to be made unilaterally by the physician or the health care team. One reason for this change was the general acceptance of a criticism made against the older paternalistic approach. Robert Veatch is one of the strongest critics of medical paternalism. In 1973, he wrote an influential article in which he attacked what he called the "generalization of expertise."[3] By this he meant the tendency of health care professionals, especially physicians, to assume that their considerable expertise in medicine gave them expertise as well in ethics and in determining correct human values for their patients. Physicians are trained to make medical decisions, he said (and I will argue that this includes decisions that a treatment is medically futile), but not necessarily to make decisions about what patients ought to do with respect to the values they cherish. To assume they could was a fallacy, the fallacy of generalization of expertise. This criticism of paternalism has been generally accepted in medical ethics and recently in American law. Though it is quite true that patient autonomy cannot stand as an absolute value in automatic preference to all others, a point being made with increasing frequency especially in the context of allocation of medical resources, the importance of autonomy is well recognized. Legally and morally, the patient is to be seen as more than a disease to be treated. The patient is also a person who makes decisions and whose values count. This change has, I think, brought with it a reduction in the automatic technological imperative that preceded it. Because physicians realize that patients and surrogates must enter into the decision-making process, physicians are now more apt to hesitate before going ahead with treatment. Perhaps ironically, the emphasis on patient autonomy has led to a situation in which physicians have begun in some cases to ignore their patients' desires to continue aggressive treatment.

A second cause of the shift from cases in which providers insist on treating and patients or families refuse treatment, to cases in which providers want to stop and families or patients insist on continuing, is the ongoing increase in medical knowledge and development of outcomes assessment. Health care providers are becoming more aware that certain procedures that initially showed great promise may not always be appropriate. This has quite properly contributed to a hesitation in performing procedures that physicians and nurses know will do little or no real good.

The third cause of the shift is more problematic. Restrictions have been placed on health care resources. In the current market-based approach to payment and insurance, hospitals often take serious losses by continuing treatment that family members wish but physicians consider unwarranted. Payment schemes such as diagnosis-related groups have resulted in major hospital losses in some cases of this type. Physicians naturally defend the fiscal viability of the hospitals in which they work. And hospitals and health maintenance organizations (HMOs) put pressure on physicians not to treat needlessly, because the hospitals or HMOs will take a loss if the cost of treatment exceeds the amount of repayment. Capitation schemes and other payment plans that penalize physicians who treat "too much" further increase this disincentive to treat. Clearly, this is a different financial incentive system from the one that formerly prevailed and that rewarded physicians for continuing aggressive treatment.

The issue of medical futility is thus important because more and more cases of conflict concern it. Physicians are arguing against treatment that patients or families want, and they are making the argument on the basis of medical futility.

A court case in Minnesota is typical. It has been called "a case of *Cruzan*-in-reverse."[4] Hennepin County Medical Center went to court seeking to turn off Helga Wanglie's respirator and withdraw artificial nutrition. Like Nancy Cruzan, Mrs. Wanglie was in a persistent vegetative state. Her care was paid for by Medicare and an HMO, so the hospital was not losing money. Rather, it claimed that the treatment was medically inappropriate, although its explicit legal claim was that Mrs. Wanglie's husband, Oliver, ought not to be the decision maker in the case. He was insisting on continuing the treatment, arguing this on the basis of his and her

Lutheran beliefs, and existing evidence suggests that Mrs. Wanglie herself would have wanted it continued as well. District Court Judge Patricia Belois decided that Mr. Wanglie was the proper decision maker. The hospital did not appeal and continued life-sustaining treatment. Mrs. Wanglie died 3 days later, on July 4, 1991. The case, discussed in greater detail later in this book, raises very difficult questions.

The Concept of Medical Futility

Let us now turn to the issue of medical futility itself. What is medical futility, and what are criteria should be used for determining that a treatment is medically futile?

Medical futility characterizes treatments that are of no medical benefit to the patient. Such treatments are contrary to the standard of medical care. Once a treatment has been categorized as medically futile, physicians must withhold or withdraw it, regardless of the wishes of the patient or surrogate. Doing so is a medical decision, not an ethical one, and depends on the proper application of medical expertise. Physicians, not ethicists or patients or their families, apply the criteria of medical futility in individual cases.

This meaning has, I am convinced, been the customary one, although it is not precise. The term is used in policies regarding forgoing treatment and seems to refer generally to treatments that doctors need not give.[5] Policies may say simply that physicians need not provide medically futile treatment.

Besides medically futile treatments, there are humanly futile treatments, including morally extraordinary or optional treatments that some patients consider useless (or "futile") for themselves but that other patients choose to undergo—for example, chemotherapy associated with a 25% chance of a 2-year remission. My topic here is what I think the term *medical futility* ought to mean.

I mentioned earlier Veatch's criticism of the generalization of expertise.[6] This criticism does not imply that health care professionals have no expertise whatsoever. Physicians are not reduced to giving their patients a list of options and a bibliography of articles in the *New England Journal of Medicine* and *Annals of Internal Medicine* and telling them to go home, read up on their conditions, and come back with choices of treatment. Physicians, nurses, physicians' assistants, and other health care professionals are still the experts in medicine and health care, and decisions can be made without consulting the patient or the patient's surrogate.

I like to use a silly case to make this clear. If I go to a dialysis center with a head cold and demand dialysis as treatment, offer $1000 in cash, insist that I am an autonomous person, quote from the literature against paternalism and the generalization of expertise, and threaten to sue if the center does not do what I want, the physician is still required ethically and legally to refuse my request. As a patient, I do not have any idea of what I am talking about. Medical expertise must override my silly request. My demand contradicts the standard of care. There is no need to refer me to another physician or nurse who might (illegally and unethically) comply with my request. The dialysis center must simply tell me that dialysis is no treatment for my cold and send me away (unless there is reason to suspect I might be psychotic and self-destructive, I suppose, and in need of psychiatric observation).

Similarly, physicians have no obligation to give medically futile treatment to any patient. If the treatment is medically futile, doctors simply do not give it. They are not obliged to inform the patient or ask the patient's permission or that of the family. This applies to cardiopulmonary resuscitation, antibiotic therapy, and all sorts of treatment that in other circumstances might be warranted but in this case are medically futile.

Criteria for Determining Medical Futility

It is clear that criteria for determining medical futility are crucial. But are these criteria within the purview of medicine, ethics, or both?

The following analogy, though not perfect, might help here. The expertise needed to determine that a patient has died is that of the physician. In a case in which cardiopulmonary function is being maintained by machines after brain dysfunction has occurred, the expertise is that of the neurologist. The neurologist runs tests to determine whether the criteria for brain death have been met, and if they have been—if total brain death has occurred—the patient is declared dead. The fact that relatives say that the patient has not yet died because they can see breathing is irrelevant. No further treatment is given. The decision is a medical one.

However, what *kind* of brain death indicates that the patient has died was not and is not determined purely on medical grounds. Society has decided that only total brain death indicates that a person is dead. The arguments that irreversibly comatose persons have already died have been rejected. The cessation of all higher brain function is not enough, it has been said, to allow one to declare a person to be dead. People do not want to bury breathing individuals, and they do not want to stop them from breathing and then bury them. This decision was an ethical and social one, not a medical one, though of course medical professionals had an important role to play in the discussion that led to the decision. Now that the criteria are ethically and legally established, doctors are the people who apply them. Doctors decide on the proper tests to use to determine whether a person is "brain-dead." But the establishment of the *kind* of brain dysfunction that indicates death—that is, the establishment of the kinds of criteria used to determine that death has occurred—involves social, legal, and ethical decisions, not purely medical decisions. This becomes even clearer when one recalls that there is still some discussion in the United States, largely in the context of organ procurement, concerning whether anencephalic patients and possibly individuals who are irreversibly comatose should be added to the ranks of the truly dead. No one suggests that the American Academy of Neurology can by itself decree this kind of change.

The same applies to the issue of medical futility. Once a treatment is determined by the physician to be medically futile, the physician must not offer it or continue it. But the determination of the kinds of treatment that are to be included in this category—that is, the determination of the kinds of criteria that must be met before medical futility can be declared—is a societal, ethical, and legal issue, not a purely medical one.

What then are the criteria proposed for determining that a treatment is medically futile? The best list of possible criteria is, in my judgment, that presented by Stuart J. Youngner in a 1988 article.[7] He suggested four possible criteria:

First, a treatment is clearly medically futile if it will fail in strictly physiological terms. The dialysis will not clear the blood, the vasopressor will not increase the blood pressure, electrical cardioversion will not start the heart, arrhythmia control will not stop the fibrillation. No one disagrees with this criterion. In such circumstances, physicians must refuse to perform the procedure, regardless of patient or surrogate requests. The procedure is, in this case, contrary to the standard of medical care. It is medically futile.

Second, a treatment might be called futile if it works in the direct or local physiological sense but does not postpone death for even a very short time. The cardioversion does start the heart, but the heart stops again almost immediately, and this occurs each time this procedure is done. The dialysis does clear the blood, but because the patient is immediately moribund from another cause, the dialysis is in fact irrelevant to the treatment for the patient's underlying disease. Now there is some question about what counts as immediate dying. If a ventilator will keep a dying patient alive for an extra day or two, but not longer, is use of it medically futile? If intubation or other intensive care unit procedures will not reverse or even significantly affect the patient's death spiral but will postpone death for a day or two, can the physician refuse a surrogate's request to intubate, on the grounds that intubation would violate the standard of medical care? There is no consensus yet about the definition of immediate dying. I would argue that dying in 2 or 3 days is immediate dying—hence the procedure in this case is medically futile. On the other hand, I would probably not consider death in 2 weeks or more immediate; in such a case, physicians could not unilaterally refuse a patient's or surrogate's request for treatment. The intervening time of delay is less certain to me, and there is no clarity in this regard in ethics or in law, though it seems most unlikely that any legal action (lawsuit) would be successful against a physician who refused treatment when medical science clearly indicated that the treatment could not have prolonged the patient's life by as much as 2 weeks.

However, there is nearly universal agreement that treatment must be withheld or withdrawn by the physician if either of the aforementioned criteria of medical futility is met. No consent is needed by the patient. The treatment is useless in the very strictly medical sense. The decision about its uselessness is made by the medical expert.

But two other possible criteria for determining medical futility were noted by Youngner. The third is the quality-of-life criterion. What if the treatment will indeed prolong physical life for a few weeks or longer but will not lead to recovery? With treatment, perhaps the patient does not survive until discharge but does survive for a time in the hospital. Or what if the treatment does result in discharge from the hospital, but the patient's level of living is such that he or she cannot continue to carry out the basic functions of life? What about the patient in a persistent vegetative state who is maintained for many years with medical nutrition and hydration?

The fourth proposed criterion is based on probability of success. What if the physician knows only that a treatment is 75% likely not to postpone dying, 20% likely to do so, though not until discharge, and only 5% likely to lead to discharge? In these cases, who makes the decision? Can this kind of futility properly be called medical futility, and can the physician therefore make a unilateral decision to withhold or withdraw treatment?

There has been considerable controversy in the literature about the question of medical futility, and the issue has received serious study over the last decade or so, though the amount of research has decreased in the last few years.[8] I myself am quite sure what the correct answer is, and this answer has been generally accepted.[9] The health care professional, usually the attending physician, may decide unilaterally to withhold or withdraw treatment when it is medically futile, and medical futility is based on the first two criteria I have noted and not on the last two. That is, a treatment is medically futile if the answer to either of the following two questions is no:

First, will the treatment do, in the immediate, local physiological sense, what it is intended to do? If the answer is no, the treatment is medically futile and must not be given.

Second, if the answer to the first question is yes and the patient is facing imminent death, will the treatment and its resulting local physiological effect cause a postponement of physical death? If the patient is about to die and the treatment does not postpone physical death, even though it does accomplish in the local physiological sense what it is intended to do (e.g., purify the blood), the fact that physical death is not postponed even a short time means that the treatment is medically futile and should not be given. It is medically futile to treat a secondary and clinically unimportant illness in a patient facing imminent death from another cause.

There is, of course, one exception to this. Treatment that relieves pain or other patient discomfort is not futile simply because it does not postpone physical death. With this exception, however, the two questions just presented can serve to define medical futility. Treatment that is futile for other reasons is not medically futile in this sense, and the decision to withhold or stop it must be made only after consultation with the patient or surrogate and only with his or her approval. Perhaps I want to be kept alive to see the Red Sox beat the Yankees even though I know I will never leave the hospital. This reason may appeal only to someone from Massachusetts, but I am, and it does appeal to me. Or perhaps a patient wants to live until after the wedding of a son or daughter; to most of us, this reason would seem a valid reason for resuscitation, even if the patient is virtually certain to die before leaving the hospital. Or perhaps a surrogate wants to continue treatment for religious reasons, or even out of fear or guilt. Such reasons do not appeal to me at all. But the consensus in the United States is that in such cases, treatment cannot be called medically futile, and the decision to withhold or withdraw treatment cannot be made unilaterally by the physician, the health care team, or the hospital.

The other criteria that have been proposed should be rejected as bases for medical futility, that is, as bases for the conclusion that physicians must unilaterally refuse to perform the procedure. As I have noted, some argue that medical futility can be determined as well on the basis of small probability of success and/or the basis of society's agreement that even a medically successful outcome is not humanly beneficial.[10] This set of criteria would enable physicians unilaterally to withhold or stop a treatment if it had a minimal (perhaps less than 1%) chance of success and/or if the medically successful outcome was one that most would not want for themselves (perhaps a persistent vegetative state).

The "and/or" in the last paragraph is important. These two criteria could be conjunctive or disjunctive: both or either of the criteria could be required to be met. There is a major difference. If the criteria are conjunctive (if both must be fulfilled), artificial nutrition and hydration for most patients in a persistent vegetative state would not meet the criteria for medical futility. The treatment might be said to yield an outcome that most of us (the "reasonable person standard") would consider to be humanly undesirable. But the odds of achieving this medically successful outcome are great. With this conjunctive use of the proposed criteria, surrogates would still be able to decide—not the physicians. But if the criteria are disjunctive—that is, if either would suffice as a basis for determining the medical futility of a proposed treatment—physicians could unilaterally choose to withdraw artificial nutrition in the case of patients like Helga Wanglie or Nancy Cruzan, because the "reasonable person" would have decided that the outcome was not truly beneficial. And it is even possible that with the disjunctive use of these criteria, I might not be able to see the Red Sox play or a parent might not see a child's wedding.

Criteria based on probability of success and societal determination of benefit ought not to be used to determine whether a treatment is medically futile. Physicians should not make unilateral decisions to withhold or with-draw treatment on this basis, notwithstanding recommendations in the literature. Patients and families should be able to decide whether to forgo a treatment with small probability of success and/or associated with poor quality of life as a result of success.

There is an area, however, where change is likely to be made in the future. Pressures for cost containment will likely lead to refusal by insurers to pay for certain treatments that have low probability of success and/or for which the outcome is one that most consider to be of no real benefit. Americans may quite properly decide that certain treatments of this kind must not be covered by Medicare or Medicaid. And private insurers may rightly offer varying policies, some of which do not cover certain treatments of this type. But this is not a question of medical futility; it is a question of allocation of resources.

Problems With This Restrictive Approach

The approach I have proposed to determine medical futility—an approach that has gained general support in the United States—is very restrictive. Most treatments that medical providers rightly and humanely want to stop will not fit into this notion of medical futility. Some families will continue to demand aggressive therapy for extremely sick patients whom such procedures will keep alive but will never truly benefit.

Physicians are often disturbed, even angered, by such requests. Why should patients and families think themselves capable of making these decisions? In the American context, part of the answer comes from the fact that for many years, many physicians and health care institutions supported a technological imperative: if a treatment that could prolong a patient's life is available, that treatment ought to be tried, regardless of the quality of the outcome or the probability of success. In the American retrospective-payment (fee-for-service) context—in which the more a doctor or hospital did, the more profit was obtained—patients and families often found themselves unable to persuade health care providers to stop treatment. In all the early related court decisions in the United States, families asked that treatments be withdrawn and hospitals or physicians refused to do so.

Gradually, the law and the ethics changed to allow patients and surrogates to make these choices. The Patient Self-Determination Act, advance directives, and state laws supporting them added and still add to this shift in decision-making authority from doctors to patients. A social sense concerning which treatments ought be done and which forgone has not emerged. Unlike many other nations, the United States has fostered this ethos of individual choice. Individuals ought to be able to receive what they want. Today's physicians and health care institutions are quite right to question the insistence by patients and surrogates that patients receive inappropriate treatments that are often very costly and are at best unlikely to benefit them. But it is important to recognize that the social context for this is one that American medicine has supported and still supports. Other social contexts, in which a general society-wide vision of proper care prevails, and in which access to health care is guaranteed by and regulated by governments or other public bodies, provide to a better extent a basis for decision making at a higher, civic level. In these other contexts, individuals are less apt to feel they have a right to anything they ask for. I fear that only systemic changes in American medicine will end the medical futility debate.

Reducing Demand for Inappropriate Treatment
There are, of course, options that can be tried to reduce patient demand for inappropriate but not medically futile treatments. Some of these would, however, require the kind of systemic change America has thus far rejected. I can think of nine options.

First, any national health insurance will quite rightly not cover such treatments. In a good national health care system, hospitals and providers also will be specifically told that they need not give such treatments to patients who cannot pay for them. Unfortunately, American abhorrence of government-mandated, single-payer universal coverage makes such an alternative unlikely in the near future.

Second, private insurance companies, medical care organizations, preferred provider organizations, HMOs, and the like may also quite rightly refuse to pay for these treatments, although the legal implications of hospitals refusing to treat would be unclear without federal or state statutory indemnification. But because private insurers are ethically and legally required to tell their clients what treatments they will and will not pay for, and because American health insurance is largely private and highly competitive, insurance companies are unlikely to refuse to cover inappropriate treatments. If one insurer told potential clients it would not pay for treatment that another covered, the former might be at a disadvantage in a market in which clients want access to all possible medical care.

Third, hospitals could establish public policies against doing this or that treatment. A hospital might say, "We do not treat patients who are in a persistent vegetative state, because we believe the resources should go to our well-baby clinic instead." That is not a medical policy in the strict sense; rather, it is a social ethical decision based on a wide range of factors including, but not limited to, the strictly medical. Hospitals are unlikely to take this approach, given possible damage to public image.

Fourth, hospitals or individual physicians can always go to court to try to get a guardian who will agree to the patient's forgoing the inadvisable treatment. A judge is most unlikely to rule in the hospital's or physician's favor, however, unless it can be shown that the surrogate is unfit because of a conflict of interest or that the treatment is not only unreasonable but actively harmful to the patient—which, with proper pain relief, should never be the case.[11]

Fifth, early review can often help reduce the number of cases of inappropriate treatment. If primary care physicians take the time to speak with their patients about these issues, many of these patients will opt against inappropriate treatment and perhaps leave advance directives regarding it. It is important to note that physicians act ethically when they advise patients and surrogates against procedures that offer little benefit. Health care providers are rightly expected by patients to give such advice. They are not supposed to behave as neutral observers and offer a list of options.

Sixth, some time spent with the family can be of great help. It takes time for families to let go. Hospital personnel should try to keep families well informed of the deteriorating condition of patients. If staff members tell a family on Monday that they have great hope that a series of diagnostic procedures will suggest a solution, but they never tell the family that in most cases the solution does not work, it is hardly surprising if on Tuesday, when told there is no hope, family members are unable to let their loved one die.

Seventh, general education of the public is important. I am convinced that the medical community does significant harm with all its competitive advertising. People are continually told only about the miracles that occur in hospitals. They naturally expect that another miracle is always possible. And there is the very problematic fact that medicine is not and cannot be an exact science. Stories often appear in the popular media (and are told in hospital shows on television) about patients whom doctors gave up on but who survived and even thrived. People naturally want that chance for themselves.

Eighth, living wills and durable powers of attorney may help families follow the expressed wishes of dying patients to forgo unreasonable life-sustaining treatment.

Ninth, it is always correct for a physician or other provider to withdraw from a case if the treatment demanded is against his or her conscience, but the provision, as always, is that some other provider will agree to care for the patient, which is unlikely in this kind of situation.

A 10th "option" was suggested by one physician, who commented that families might be dissuaded from unreasonable treatment if intensive care units included coin-operated ventilators!

Conclusion

In the light of recent legal decisions and of the present American ethical consensus, physicians and other providers ought not to declare medical futility when a treatment prolongs the patient's life by any humanly significant length. Such treatment may well be inadvisable, silly, too costly, or even degrading. But this kind of quality-of-life decision should be made by the patient or the surrogate, not unilaterally by the physician. It is not strictly a medical decision, but a decision that includes ethical and social dimensions. Perhaps in the future, American support for individual decision-making in health care will be balanced by a recognition of the needs of society and of the common good. But until systemic change occurs, the decision belongs to the patient and not to the physician.

Notes

[1] *Cruzan v Missouri Department of Health,* 497 US 261 (1990).

[2] Two exceptions are so rare that this is almost an absolute right. There have been some exceptions made in the case of a parent (usually a mother) of a young child, but many argue that this is sexist, and the exception has not been imposed for many years. Exceptions are

sometimes made concerning pregnant women whose fetuses might live to be born alive, but this is medically rare.

[3]Robert M. Veatch, "Generalization of Expertise," *Hastings Center Studies* 1:29–40, 1973.

[4]"Courting the Issues: Decisions in Minnesota and Missouri," *Hospital Ethics* 7:2–5, 1991.

[5]This seems to be the usage of the term in the hospital policy on forgoing treatment, which simply states: "If requested treatment is medically futile or non-beneficial, it need not be provided" (p. 4). But the coupling of the term *medically futile* with the less precise term *non-beneficial* shows a lack of detailed development of the meaning. Indeed, the policy goes on to say that physicians who refuse to give such treatment, like those who object on ethical or religious grounds, may withdraw treatment but must transfer the patient to the care of another. The meaning of medical futility that I am arguing for here would neither require not permit such a transfer.

[6]Veatch, "Generalization of Expertise," 29–40.

[7]Stuart J. Youngner, "Who Defines Futility?" *JAMA* 260:2094–5, 1988.

[8]In addition to Youngner's article, already cited, articles include Leslie J. Blackhall, "Must We Always Use CPR?" *New England Journal of Medicine* 317:1281–5, 1987 (Blackhall gives more latitude to physicians in terms of making unilateral decisions than I believe is appropriate); Tom Tomlinson and Howard Brody, "Ethics and Communication in Do-Not-Resuscitate Orders," *New England Journal of Medicine* 318:43–6, 1988 (these authors make helpful distinctions between medical futility and quality-of-life futility); Donald J. Murphy, "Do-Not-Resuscitate Orders: Time for Reappraisal in Long-Term-Care Institutions," *JAMA* 260:2098–101, 1988 (Murphy argues that physicians may unilaterally write a do-not-resuscitate order when the future quality of life will be low [p. 2100], a position I do not accept); Troyen A. Brennan, "Incompetent Patients With Limited Care in the Absence of Family Consent. A Study of Socioeconomic and Clinical Variables," *Annals of Internal Medicine* 109:819–25, 1988; Philip J. Boyle, "DNR and the Elderly," *Issues in Health Care,* December 1988; John D. Lantos et al, "The Illusion of Futility in Clinical Practice," *American Journal of Medicine* 87:81–4, 1989; John J. Paris, Robert K. Crone, and Frank Reardon, "Physicians' Refusal of Requested Treatment: The Case of Baby L," *New England Journal of Medicine* 322:1012–5, 1990; Daniel Callahan, "Medical Futility, Medical Necessity: The-Problem-Without-A-Name," *Hastings Center Report* 21:30–5, 1991 (Callahan's approach is similar to mine); Mildred Z. Solomon, "How Physicians Talk About Futility: Making Words Mean Too Many Things," *Journal of Law, Medicine & Ethics* 21:231–7, 1993; Laurence J. Schneiderman, Kathy Faber-Langendoen, and Nancy S. Jecker, "Beyond Futility to an Ethic of Care," *American Journal of Medicine* 96:110–4, 1994; Stuart J. Youngner, "Applying Futility: Saying No Is Not Enough," *Journal of the American Geriatrics Society* 42:887–9, 1994; Judy Laffey, "Bioethical Principles and Care-Based Ethics in Medical Futility," *Cancer Practice* 4:41–6, 1996; "Medical Futility in End-of-Life Care: Report of the Council on Ethical and Judicial Affairs," *JAMA* 281:937–41, 1999; Amir Halevy and Baruch A. Brody, "Medical Futility in End-of-Life Care," *JAMA* 282:1331–2, 1999; and Paul R. Helft, Mark Siegler, and John Lantos, "The Rise and Fall of the Futility Movement," *New England Journal of Medicine* 343:293–6, 2000.

[9]This approach to medical futility is followed in the draft of a proposed statement by the Ethics Committee of the Society of Critical Care Medicine (draft of July 8, 1996). It is also implied in the Council on Ethical and Judicial Affairs of the American Medical Association, "Medical Futility in End-of-Life Care," *JAMA* 281:937–41, 1999. That published statement does not suggest that quality-of-life decisions may be made unilaterally by physicians. See also Paul R. Helft, Mark Siegler, and John Lantos, "The Rise and Fall of the Futility

Movement," *New England Journal of Medicine* 343:293–6, 2000. The authors note that the futility debate has largely died out because the attempt to expand the criteria has been medically, legally, and ethically unsuccessful. The authors also note that attempts at objectifying and quantifying outcomes of treatments have failed, thus making it difficult, if not impossible, to base decisions about quality of life and probability of success on clear and certain medical criteria. Attempts at designing medical futility policies have been process based and have rejected any unilateral decisions by physicians, which of course is exactly what medical futility is supposed to enable. The approach suggested here is also supported in John D. Lantos et al, "The Illusion of Futility in Clinical Practice," *American Journal of Medicine* 87:81–4, 1989; these authors argue that patients are best able to make decisions of this kind because their personal values and goals differ.

[10]These criteria are proposed in Lawrence J. Schneiderman, Nancy S. Jecker, and Albert R. Jonsen, "Medical Futility: Its Meaning and Ethical Implications," *Annals of Internal Medicine* 112:949–54, 1990. These authors argue that either a very small probability of medical success (less than 1%–3%; no successes in the last 100 cases) or an outcome that does not benefit the patient as a whole (the treatment only prolongs the life of an unconscious patient, or the treatment maintains life but the patient remains dependent on intensive medical care) is a sufficient warrant for declaring a treatment medically futile. They wish these criteria to be independent; meeting either one is enough. They propose that nutritional support for a patient in a persistent vegetative state be considered medically futile and that physicians withhold or withdraw such support, regardless of the wishes of the patient or the family (p. 950). If medical care does not offer patients the opportunity to achieve any of life's goals, physicians must refuse to give it, regardless of the wishes of patients or surrogates (pp. 949, 952–3).

[11]The Wanglie case is one example. See also Paul R. Helft, Mark Siegler, and John Lantos, "The Rise and Fall of the Futility Movement," *New England Journal of Medicine* 343:293–6, 2000 at p. 295; these authors quote J. F. Daar ("Medical Futility and Implications for Physician Autonomy," *American Journal of Law and Medicine* 21:221–40, 1995) as saying that almost every court case of this kind has been resolved in favor of the patient. They list one notable exception *(Gilgunn v Massachusetts General Hospital),* but that was a jury decision, not a court ruling.

Selected Bibliography

Ackerman F: The significance of a wish. Hastings Cent Rep 1991;21:27–9. An argument that Helga Wanglie's treatment should be chosen by her husband.

Blackhall LJ: Must we always use CPR? N Engl J Med 1987;317:1281–5.

Boyle PJ: DNR and the elderly. Issues in Health Care, December 1988.

Brennan TA: Incompetent patients with limited care in the absence of family consent. A study of socioeconomic and clinical variables. Ann Intern Med 1988;109:819–25.

Callahan D: Medical futility, medical necessity: the-problem-without-a-name. Hastings Cent Rep 1991;21:30–5.

Capron AM: Medical futility: strike two. Hastings Cent Rep 1994;24:42–3.

Capron AM: Abandoning a waning life. Hastings Cent Rep 1995;25:24–6.

Cranford RE: Helga Wanglie's ventilator. Hastings Cent Rep 1991;21:23–4. A general description of this case.

Kapp MB: Futile medical treatment: a review of the ethical arguments and legal holdings. J Gen Intern Med 1994;9:170–7.

Kelly DF: Critical Care Ethics: Treatment Decisions in American Hospitals. Kansas City,

MO: Sheed & Ward, 1991.

Morreim EH: Profoundly diminished life: the casualties of coercion. Hastings Cent Rep 1994;24:33–42. An argument against the use of the word *futility* to enable physicians to make unilateral moral decisions.

Murphy DJ: Do-not-resuscitate orders: time for reappraisal in long-term-care institutions. JAMA 1988;260:2098–101.

Paris JJ, Crone RK, Reardon F: Physicians' refusal of requested treatment: the case of Baby L. N Engl J Med 1990;322:1012–5.

Rie MA: The limits of a wish. Hastings Cent Rep 1991;21:24–7. An argument that the treatment for Helga Wanglie should be stopped.

Schneiderman LJ, Jecker NS, Jonsen AR: Medical futility: its meaning and ethical implications. Ann Intern Med 1990;112:949–54. These authors argue that the term *medical futility* applies to all treatments that are very unlikely to be successful or that, if successful, lead to a very poor outcome. Their argument is the most articulate thus far in defense of the position I oppose.

Solomon MZ: How physicians talk about futility: making words mean too many things. J Law Med Ethics 1993;21:231–7.

Tomlinson T, Brody H: Ethics and communication in do-not-resuscitate orders. N Engl J Med 1988;318:43–6. These authors make very helpful distinctions between medical futility and quality-of-life futility.

Youngner SJ: Who defines futility? JAMA 1988;260:2094–5. A very helpful description of possible criteria to use for determining medical futility.

Multinational Perspective on Treatment of the Three Patients

Description of the Cases

David Crippen, MD

To examine the problem of futility in intensive care, the editors asked a multinational sampling of critical care physicians to describe how they would treat their critically ill patients. We formulated three patient cases based on actual patients, with any distinguishing characteristics obscured to maintain confidentiality. We queried, through electronic mail, a number of the critical care physicians subscribed to the multinational critical care electronic list CCM-L (http://ccm-l.med.edu). Before the Internet, contacting physicians around the world would have been a lengthy and laborious process. In this instance, it was accomplished in a week.

The cases illustrated three clinical scenarios. Patient A is a critically ill and unstable patient who is predicted to benefit from short-term critical care. He receives aggressive care with a strong potential to reverse organ system insufficiency and enable him to become a productive member of society once more. Patient B is a critically ill patient who may or may not benefit from the application of critical care technology and who is treated aggressively. Subsequently, he stops benefiting from treatment and becomes dependent on life support. A critical deadlock is reached: the patient's family desires to maintain life-support systems indefinitely, with negligible predicted benefit, and physicians desire to stop the same care because it will not return the patient to sentient life. Patient C is a moribund patient with multiple organ system failure who desires the use of life-support systems despite the expressed opinion of critical care physicians that such care will do nothing but increase his discomfort during the inevitable dying process.

We asked the critical care physicians to respond to two questions:

Question 1: How would you actually treat each patient with the resources currently available to you and in the context of existing sociopolitical pressures?

Question 2: How would you treat each patient if you had unlimited resources and had unlimited authority to use them?

To the best of our knowledge, this kind of clinical evaluation has never been done until now.

A set of questions at the end of each clinical presentation stimulated qualitative and quantitative assessments by a multinational group of practicing critical care physicians. These questions were organized into the following four groups: 1) What resources are available in different parts of the world for aggressive treatment of critically ill patients? How are these resources prioritized? 2) How do physicians around the world predict which patients will respond to salvage treatment, if indeed attempts at prediction are made? And during the course of treatment, how do physicians ascertain the point of diminishing returns, when detriment exceeds benefit? 3) How do physicians around the world differentiate between medically-futile and medically inappropriate treatment in a care plan? 4) How do physicians around the world say no to continuation of aggressive and invasive care, if indeed they do?

The fundamental issue in the examination of these three cases and how the patients' care relates to physicians' abilities to provide critical care services lies in a qualitative dissonance between Patient B and Patient C. Patient B has some reasonable chance of benefit, but there is a potential point of diminishing returns. Aggressive care continued after that point has been reached constitutes medically inappropriate care, even if it is technically not medically futile. Patient C cannot be saved by any means and should be denied critical care on the basis of medical futility, even if he or his family desires it.

Here are the patients:

Patient A

Patient A is a 57-year-old man with a history of mild hypertension, for which he irregularly takes medication. He developed chest pain and was seen in an outlying community hospital emergency department (ED), where he was found to have electrocardiographic changes compatible with myocardial injury. He was taken to the cardiac catheterization laboratory for rescue angioplasty, and during the procedure he developed a malignant arrhythmia and experienced cardiac arrest. During the advanced cardiac life-support protocol, he aspirated gastric contents while undergoing intubation. Ultimately, a functional cardiac rhythm was restored, and he was transferred to the cardiac care unit, intubated. Over the next 3 days, he developed aspiration pneumonia, sepsis, acute respiratory distress syndrome, and renal failure, and he was transferred to the medical intensive care unit (ICU) by helicopter because the referring facility "couldn't handle him."

On arrival, the patient is obtunded and only grimaces in response to painful stimuli. He is intubated and is receiving mechanical ventilation with an FIO_2 of 100% and a positive end-expiratory pressure (PEEP) of 5 cm H_2O. The patient's arterial oxygen saturation (SaO_2) is 88%. His blood pressure is 78/25 mm Hg, and his extremities are cool. His urine output is 5 mL/h. He is receiving normal saline at an infusion rate of 75 mL/h. He has been given two doses of a first-generation cephalosporin. No vasopressors or inotropic agents are being infused. The patient has no health insurance.

His chest radiograph shows extensive bilateral infiltrates. An electrocardiogram (ECG) shows normal sinus rhythm (NSR) with a rate of 130 beats/min, multifocal premature ventricular contractions, and an inferior injury pattern. His hemoglobin level is 15 g/dL, and the white blood cell (WBC) count is 18,000/mm³. An electrolyte panel is normal except for a blood urea nitrogen (BUN) concentration of 61 mg/dL (22 mmol/L) and a serum creatinine concentration of 6.1 mg/dL (539 μmol/L). A coagulation profile shows a prothrombin time (PT) of 21 seconds and a partial thromboplastin time (PTT) of 69 seconds. No heparin is being infused. Liver function enzyme levels are increased, and the amylase level is 347 U/L. Cardiac enzyme and troponin levels are increased.

Patient B

Patient B is an 88-year-old man with a history of diabetes, hypertension, peripheral vascular disease, atherosclerotic heart disease, chronic renal insufficiency, chronic obstructive pulmonary disease, and dementia. His medications include subcutaneous insulin, two antihypertensives, aspirin, and nitroglycerin paste (applied every 6 hours). He receives 24-hour oxygen via nasal cannula, and his baseline SaO_2 is reported to be 92%. He resides in a skilled nursing home.

He was transferred to the ED after staff noticed that he was febrile and the urine output from his Foley catheter had decreased to nothing. In the ED, he was hypotensive and tachycardic, with no appreciable urine output, and he was unresponsive. His SaO_2 while he was receiving oxygen via nasal cannula was 78%. His relatives were called, and they stated that they wanted everything done. Accordingly, he was intubated and mechanical ventilation was begun. A central line was placed, and after fluid resuscitation, his blood pressure increased to 90/50 mm Hg. He was transferred to the medical ICU.

He is thin, cachectic, and deconditioned and has large decubiti over his sacrum. He responds to painful stimuli by grimacing. His blood pressure is 80/37 mm Hg. Heart rate is 140 beats/min in sinus tachycardia. With an FIO_2 of 100% and a PEEP of 5 cm H_2O, his SaO_2 is 88%. His extremities are cool, and his urine output is less than 5 mL/h. The patient is receiving normal saline at an infusion rate of 75 mL/h. He has been given two doses of a first-generation cephalosporin. No vasopressors or inotropic agents are being infused.

His chest radiograph shows extensive bilateral infiltrates. An ECG shows NSR with a rate of 140 beats/min, multifocal premature ventricular contractions, and other nonspecific changes. His hemoglobin level is 15 g/dL, and the WBC count is 38,000/mm^3. An electrolyte panel shows a serum potassium concentration of 5.9 mEq/L, BUN level of 91 mg/dL (32 mmol/L), and serum creatinine level of 8.1 mg/dL (716 µmol/L).

Ultimately, the patient develops fluid overload and pulmonary edema during volume loading, and large doses of diuretics do not promote diuresis. Blood gas measurements indicate significant metabolic acidosis.

There is no living will, nor are there advance directives on the chart. The patient is clearly incompetent to voice his wishes. His relatives are contacted again and the situation is explained to them in detail, including his grave prognosis. They respond that they want everything done because they believe that the patient will improve, as he has in the past, if aggressive care is continued. The patient has no health insurance.

Patient C

Patient C is a 42-year-old man with an extensive ethanol dependency history and acquired immunodeficiency syndrome (AIDS), for which he has been intermittently followed in a free clinic when he chooses to attend. He has a history of noncompliance with his AIDS medications. He drinks a liter of hard liquor a day and has never shown any interest in rehabilitation. He called the ambulance after an episode of vomiting blood and was taken to the ED for evaluation.

In the ED, he is seen to be thin, cachectic, deconditioned, and clearly jaundiced. He is 6 ft 1 in (1.85 m) tall and weighs 92 lb (42 kg). He is intermittently vomiting gross blood into a bucket. His blood pressure is 90/36 mm Hg and his heart rate is 140 beats/min in sinus tachycardia. While the patient is being given 100% oxygen via a nonrebreather mask, his SaO$_2$ is 88%. He has no urine output from his Foley catheter. He is oozing blood from every orifice.

His chest radiograph shows extensive bilateral infiltrates. An ECG shows NSR with a rate of 140 beats/min, multifocal premature ventricular contractions, and other nonspecific changes. His hemoglobin level is 4 g/dL, and the WBC count is 34,000/mm^3. An electrolyte panel shows a serum sodium level of 115 mEq/L, serum potassium level of 6.2 mEq/L, BUN concentration of 174 mg/dL (62 mmol/L), and serum creatinine level of 13.1 mg/dL (1202 μmol/L). A coagulation profile shows a PT of 40 seconds and a PTT of more than 200 seconds. Liver function enzyme levels are dramatically increased. His total bilirubin level is 28 mg/dL (479 μmol/L).

He is lucid, has some paranoid ideation, answers questions, and gives a history. When told of his moribund condition, he states emphatically that he wants everything done. He further states that he believes a "miracle" will save him if very aggressive care is continued. When options are read to him, he desires them all: intubation, mechanical ventilation, vasoactive infusions, and dialysis. There are no living relatives. He has no health insurance.

South Africa

Richard Burrows, MB, BCh

Patient A

Upwards of 50% of patients are refused admission to our unit, because of a lack of resources to deal with the patient load. Furthermore, because of the acute conditions of the patients admitted, mortality rates are often around 40%. The total budget for the hospital is in the region of US$26 million. This is a 750-bed hospital with several outlying clinics. The intensive care unit (ICU) consists of 8 beds; there are approximately 500 cases per year. The budget of this ICU is substantially lower than that of an American ICU, where the cost of managing 100 consecutive patients can run more than US$6 million, of which more than 50% is spent on nonsurvivors.[1] It is unconscionable that in a country where human immunodeficiency virus (HIV) infection is epidemic, such funds are used for those whose chance of survival is remote. It is not only a problem in ICUs. Resources are such that, for example, patients no longer regarded as candidates for kidney trans-plantation are removed from the dialysis program. It is clear that choices must be made among patients, and there is little to be gained by emotional debates around the fact that a given patient may survive, for such can be said of any patient, no matter how sick.

No rational approach allows relatives of individual patients to decide issues of treatment under these circumstances, which are more properly addressed at a political level. Informed consent is clearly an issue, but only in terms of information regarding a medical action that is actually being proposed. The main issue in the case of Patient A is that the patient and the relatives must be informed, but it is an ethical fraud to ask them to agree to something to which they cannot agree.

In the current case, the picture is one of shock, respiratory failure, and renal failure. There is also the real possibility of hypoxic encephalopathy. A cardiac event progressed to severe multisystem failure, and the overall picture is one of rapid deterioration, to the point that dialysis and inotropes will be necessary to maintain the situation. The prognosis is grim, and the probability of death under these circumstances is extremely high.

Thus a choice must necessarily be made among patients. If this patient were to be offered the ICU bed, there is every likelihood that others with a better chance of survival would be denied treatment. The relatives would be offered a second opinion and the chance to transfer the patient to another institution, should they wish to undertake the expense.

To ask what one would do supposing resources were infinite implies that more and more resources should be expended on those patients with a vanishingly small chance of survival. However, should the patient or relatives wish to continue treatment under these circumstances, there does not seem to be any point (short of decomposition) at which the physician may insist on stopping treatment. The debate then becomes one of which inotrope to use, which antibiotic, what dialysis fluid, what fluid, and so on. In fact, the arguments themselves become infinitely numerous as the relative benefits of each treatment become negligible, and essentially unprovable. Because immortality is not possible, there will still be a point at which treatment of the underlying condition cannot be expected to achieve the goal of returning the patient to health.

Patient B

Patient B is not going to survive. At age 88 years, he presents with respiratory failure, cardiac failure, and renal failure and with preexisting disease complicated by a debilitated state. The report of the President's Commission for the Study of Ethical Problems in Medicine and Biomedical and Behavioral Research,[2] in the section entitled "Disservice of Empty Rhetoric," includes discussion of the harmful effects of using words that are little more than slogans. Phrases such as *right to die* and *right to life* are accepted without their meanings being questioned. Expressions such as "everything must be done" are treated no differently. The harm arises when medical staff and patients, and their relatives, have quite different concepts of what the word *everything* means. Prognostication at the end of life is notoriously uncertain, and in the face of impending death, there is an unwillingness to accept any decision not based on certainty.

For the most part, however, as in the case of this patient, dying is a process wherein the eventual outcome is certain but the point of irreversibility is not definable, and thus the decision to stop resuscitation is based on probability. There is always the possibility, however slight, that one is wrong, and it is therefore extremely stressful for both relative and physician, because the decision to stop is irrevocable. There arises a stubborn quest for certainty in predicting the outcome in order to avoid the responsibility of such a decision. Dostoyevsky pointed out that one really does not want freedom or responsibility. The living will, which is a surprisingly rare document, may simply indicate that patients too do not want to face the inevitability of death.

At a time when resuscitation was essentially nonexistent, the Hippocratic Oath was little more than a gentle hypocrisy designed more to affect the behavior of the physician than to do anything else. In the 21st century, the oath, though still important, is often little more than an invocation to press ahead and stack treatment on treatment with little or no chance of success. In this respect, "the old man's friend," pneumonia, is no longer a friend but a condition to be treated with ventilators, antibiotics, antifungals, physiotherapy, alveolar recruitment, and so on, with little thought paid to anything other than the fact that in the physiological sense, the patient is still alive and thus such treatment is achieving its goal.

There can be little doubt that Patient B has entered the dying process. There is chronic disease of the cardiovascular, respiratory, and renal systems. He is cachectic and deconditioned with decubital ulcers. He is unable to maintain oxygenation, and at his advanced age, it is reasonable to presume that he has begun to die. In the face of a shortage of resources, he should not be admitted to the ICU.

What if resources were infinite? Death is still a certain end to life. In this regard, a lack of resources is often used as an excuse to avoid proceeding with treatment. In this case, it does not matter that resources are infinite. He is dying and there should be no need or duty to accede to commands that everything be done. Such demands often appear to be driven by ignorance on the one hand and fear and guilt on the other. Ignorance can be countered by information, and it is clear that relatives must be given clear and concise information. For the physician, there is the fear of legal or administrative action, a rationale of prophylaxis, or the approach of acting "just in case." Clear, full, and open discussion and a development of trust will allay most of these fears, but occasionally there is no success and it seems the issue must go to litigation, which is little more than a failure of medical practice and does nothing for the patient, because there is no guarantee that legal action will result in an outcome acceptable to anybody.

Although medical paternalism has rightly been thrown out, it does not follow that all medical decisions are paternalistic and a diagnosis of death or impending death is a medical decision.

Patient C

During testifying before the Select Committee of Parliament after the first heart transplantation, jurists insisted on a precise definition of death. Chris

Barnard testily replied, "A person is dead when the doctor says he is dead."[3] There is little evidence that anyone else wants to make the decision not to resuscitate. "The decision is not one for judicial decision but for the attending physician, in keeping with the highest traditions of his profession. It is a question peculiarly within the competence of the medical profession of what measures are appropriate to ease the passing of an irreversibly, terminally ill patient in the light of the patient's history and condition and wishes of the family."[4] The physician may in particular judge that the investment in instruments and personnel is disproportionate to the results foreseen; he or she may also judge that the techniques applied impose strain or suffering on the patient out of proportion to any expected benefits.

In order that a decision may be given effect, there must be acceptance of the fact that a decision represents an imperfect choice. Because prognosis is not a precise science and is judged against the yardstick of the certainty of death, there is an accountability to be held against a wrong decision. It is easy to understand the insistence that the patient make the decision himself or herself. The cynic would point out that having died, the patient could hardly be punished for his or her accountable action.

It has also been argued that decisions to stop treatment considered futile are merely illusions, nothing more than an attempt to put a probability score on survival, and given that certainty is nonexistent in the individual case, futility may not be invoked and the chance, however small, should be given to the patient. This approach is particularly evident in the developed world, where the medical decision to stop treatment is simply not allowed and there is no inclination to make any decision other than to stack treatment on treatment, with little regard to efficacy. In the face of death, the decision to stop treatment is irrevocable, and few physicians in the developed world seem willing to accept responsibility for such a decision, which denies the patient a chance, however small. This "stubborn quest for diagnostic certainty" flies in the face of practicality when resources are scarce. It is hardly any better when resources are plentiful.

The World Health Organization estimated that in 1999, a total of 23.3 million people were infected with HIV—10 million in South Africa, an incidence of 20%. The disease has spawned prejudices of biblical proportions. Interestingly, the prejudices are remarkably similar to the prejudices and moral panic that were part of the syphilis epidemic in the early part of the last century. The problem in South Africa is enormous, and it is far beyond the capacity of the country to respond in terms of treatment. Because resources must, by reasonable necessity, be channeled toward prevention, vaccination, and early management of the disease, there can be little argument that the management of the disease in its final stages should be little more than palliation and comfort care. Against this backdrop, treatment in the ICU vanishes to insignificance. The "miracle" would not be recovery in this patient but rather a development of reasonable treatment options and ultimate control of the disease for society as a whole. Nonetheless, Patient C is asking for a miracle.

Implicit in the argument is the notion that if the physician does not comply, he or she is playing God (an accusation often leveled at physicians) and will be held accountable. The argument can be applied to any situation in which a decision is made contrary to the wishes of another, and if it is believed that humans are made in God's image, it can be said that they play God every time they make a decision. There can be little argument that this patient is close to the end, with his multiple complications, and in the face of the shortfall of resources in this country, admitting him to the ICU cannot be justified. Care should consist only of simple medical and social measures according to his need for comfort.

If this patient is granted his wish to continue with ventilation, then the validity of claims of resource shortfalls in the developed world must be questioned. In such a case, if authorities are forced to provide a service that clearly is inappropriate, it is small wonder that third parties responsible for the service can act only by denying reimbursement or closing down on budgets. However, it does not matter that resources might be said to be infinite; even if they are, a decision will still have to be made to stop treatment at some stage. It is merely the point at which the decision is made that differs. If it is not the physician who decides, and the patient will not or is unable to come to terms with his own mortality, who must make the decision?

References

[1]Borlase BC, Baxter JT, Benotti PN, et al: Surgical intensive care unit resource use in a specialty referral hospital: I. Predictors of early death and cost implications. Surgery 1991;109:687–93.

[2]President's Commission for the Study of Ethical Problems in Medicine and Biomedical and Behavioral Research: Deciding to Forego Life-Sustaining Treatment: A Report on the Ethical, Medical and Legal Issues in Treatment Decisions. Washington, DC: U.S. Government Printing Office, 1983, pp. 24–6.

[3]Strauss SA: Doctor, Patient and the Law: A Selection of Practical Issues. Johannesburg, South Africa: Van Schaik, 1980, p. 366.

[4]Paris JJ, Reardon FE: Moral, ethical and legal issues in the intensive care unit. J Intensive Care Med 1991;6:189.

Australia

Malcolm Fisher, MD

For each patient, the answers to questions 1 and 2 are the same.

Patient A

We would admit Patient A to the intensive care unit (ICU). In addition to blood cultures, blood gas measurements, determination of electrolyte levels, and electrocardiography, we would request that echocardiograms be obtained as soon as possible. It is likely that this would be followed with some form of invasive cardiovascular monitoring. In our institution, this would involve placement of a thermodilution catheter, although an arterial catheter, which also produces thoracic blood volume and lung water results, would be of more use. If the patient was peripherally cold and shut down, we would probably commence dobutamine 200 mg in 100 mL of normal saline at about 20 mL/h before inserting the Swan-Ganz catheter.

The information given by the Swan-Ganz catheter would probably help us in two ways. If the filling pressures were high, we could take steps to lower them by administering vasodilator drugs or by using increasing doses of furosemide in an attempt to establish diuresis. The diuresis would likely be more effective if the cardiac index was greater than 2 and there was a reasonable blood pressure. Dobutamine or milrinone might be started to boost cardiac output, improve peripheral perfusion and urine output, and correct a falling base deficit. Norepinephrine would be given, if necessary, to produce a mean arterial blood pressure greater than 65 mm Hg. It would be nice to get the cardiac index above 2.5, but as a general principle, we do not like to push a diseased heart very much higher than this.

If a urine output was not established within 2 hours of admission and there was radiological evidence of increased lung water and/or peripheral edema, continuous venovenous hemofiltration would be strongly considered. The normal saline infusion would be reduced considerably. On occasion, some patients need volume. If the filling pressures and cardiac output were low, the patient would be given a trial of volume, either a crystalloid or a colloid, depending on the individual consultant's preference.

Attention would then be given to the patient's ventilation. The initial goal would be to rapidly decrease his inspired oxygen to a safe level. With a saturation of 88% and an FIO_2 of 100%, it is likely that considerable reduction in FIO_2 could be achieved without a significant deterioration in saturation. We would prefer to keep the saturation at 90% or greater. With a reasonable cardiac output established, the next task would be to establish the optimum form of ventilation for the patient and the optimum level of positive end-expiratory pressure (PEEP). The first mode of ventilation we would probably try would be inverse ratio pressure control mode (often patients like Patient A are receiving volume ventilation when they arrive at the ICU and the conversion to pressure control ventilation is associated with improvement). Once the mode of ventilation was established, a trial of PEEP would be started. Positive end-expiratory pressure would be increased to 20 cm H_2O, and if there was no significant effect on cardiac output, PEEP would be decreased in 5-cm increments about 10 minutes apart.

A cardiological opinion would be sought about the need for further angiography and for cardiac surgery. (We would want this patient's condition to improve considerably before cardiac surgery was undertaken.) Therapy would not be stopped for at least 3 days, unless signs of brain injury appeared clinically.

Patient B

In Australia, it is unlikely that Patient B would be transferred to the ICU. In our unit, the only criterion for admission is the presence of reversible disease. This patient does not have reversible disease. The first mistake was resuscitating him in the emergency department. The second mistake was taking him into the ICU. If by some mishap this patient were transferred to our ICU, there would be discussion among the ICU staff, the pulmonologist (who likely would have been the person to admit the patient), and the nursing staff caring for him, and a clear agreement would be reached that this patient would not receive dialysis or cardiopulmonary resuscitation. He would be sedated.

When there was medical and nursing consensus, we would institute immediate discussion with the relatives. If the relatives said that they wanted everything done (irrespective of the patient's insurance status or his past performances), we would tell them that we were prepared to continue for a short period and that we would like to discuss this with them on a daily basis. We would add that no additional treatments (including dialysis) would be instituted. If agreement could not be reached (it is usually not difficult to reach such an agreement with families in this country), we would then offer to obtain second opinions from any doctors they cared to name, or endeavor to have the patient transferred to an ICU that might be prepared to continue aggressive treatment.

The nursing procedures for the patient would be restricted to the minimum possible: the patient would be kept clean and comfortable, but there would be infrequent or no routine observations. It is likely that in the absence of dialysis, the patient would soon die, and we would not be unhappy if the patient's family spent time with the patient during this period, but it would be made clear to the family that if the patient's heart stopped or other complications occurred, we would not intervene. It is unlikely in these circumstances that there would be a need for unilateral withdrawal of support to facilitate bed turnover.

Patient C
We would probably offer Patient C a period of noninvasive ventilation and appropriate antibiotic therapy, but he would be informed that in our hands, the possibility of a reasonable outcome with artificial ventilation and other forms of major invasive treatment was not great and we would not institute these treatments. If he wished a second opinion, we would arrange that for him. He would be offered the option of being sedated for comfort.

United Kingdom

Anna Batchelor, MB, ChB

Patient A

In the United Kingdom, it is unlikely that angioplasty would be the first-choice treatment for a patient with signs of acute myocardial infarction. In my region of more than 2 million people, fewer than 5 of the 17 hospitals allowing acute nontriaged medical admissions have the facilities for rescue angioplasty. If it were thought that this was the appropriate treatment, the patient would have to be transferred at that stage to one of those hospitals. Very few patients are transferred from intensive care unit (ICU) to ICU by helicopter; in my area, only one helicopter is operated by the regional ambulance service, and this helicopter is more suited to primary retrieval than secondary transfer. Few hospitals have helipads. It is less time-consuming to transfer a patient by road than by helicopter if no helipads are available, because the latter type of transfer involves exporting the patient from the unit on a trolley, transferring him or her to an ambulance for the trip to the local park or open space, transferring the patient to the helicopter, flying to another park or open space, transferring the patient into another ambulance, and transferring him or her into the hospital. A marginally more suitable helicopter (bigger, but with no medical facilities) is offered by the military. However, it is not always available, and the hospital is charged for its use. The transfer team members may not be returned to their base if the helicopter is called elsewhere. Use of a helicopter from a park (i.e., a non-official landing space) may mean other emergency services are needed, such as police to control crowds and prevent injury.

As presented, Patient A has multiple organ failure with respiratory, renal, cardiovascular, hepatic, and neurological failure. My major concern at this stage would be whether this man would respond neurologically to salvage treatment. All inter-ICU transfers should be made on a consultant-to-consultant referral basis. Before accepting this patient for transfer, I would want to know what sedation he had received, if any, and what his current best responses were. At 3 days post–hypoxic-ischemic event, if the patient has abnormal brain stem responses, absent verbal response, absent withdrawal to painful stimuli, and a significantly increased serum creatinine level, he has a very poor chance of survival with or without severe disability.[1] In addition to his original insult, this patient appears to have had a continuing insult; this normally hypertensive man has hypotension. If I were not satisfied with the responses, I would get in my car and go look at the patient before agreeing to his transfer. Patients can be "dumped" on me only if I agree; in the United Kingdom, hospitals do not accept other hospitals' patients—doctors do.

If I thought he was retrievable with an acceptable neurological function, or if I thought his on-board sedation might be masking his true mental status, I would arrange his transfer. I would insist that he be appropriately resuscitated before transfer, to include administration of fluids, inotropes, and more appropriate ventilation. If his condition could not be optimized before transfer, I would refuse to accept him. If necessary, I would send out a senior trainee or consultant to supervise resuscitation and transfer; however, we are not funded for this. Interhospital transfers are audited for number, reason, and quality.

Initial resuscitation would follow standard protocol regarding airway, breathing, and circulation. His ventilation is clearly inappropriate; however, a saturation of 88% would do for now, because I suspect that once he was cardiovascularly resuscitated, this would improve. It may be spuriously low because of poor perfusion or poor cardiac output. An arterial blood gas analysis would be more accurate. Adjustment of ventilation to produce a higher mean intrathoracic pressure before cardiovascular resuscitation would be counterproductive. We would infuse fluid (a mixture of crystalloid [Hartman solution] and colloid [starch]) while inserting a triple-lumen central line and, just in case, a Swan sheath. We would assess response to fluid by measuring blood pressure, peripheral perfusion, and, it would be hoped, urine output, although there might now be established renal failure.

Inotropes, vasoconstrictors, or vasodilators would be tailored to need with, if necessary, information from a pulmonary artery catheter. Ventilation would be adjusted to produce adequate oxygenation, with CO_2 clearance as a secondary consideration; however, given that this patient has had a significant and ongoing cerebral insult, I would be loath to run his CO_2 very high. Assuming adequate resuscitation did not restore renal function, continuous venovenous hemofiltration would be commenced with 2 L/h exchanges and bicarbonate replacement solution to normalize acid-base status. Samples would be sent for microbiological analysis, and assuming a Gram stain did not reveal a significant pathogen, treatment with cefuroxime and metronidazole as first-line cover for aspiration pneumonia would be commenced. Further antibiotic or antifungal therapy would be guided by microbiological findings. Sedation would be as required; short-acting agents such as propofol and alfentanil would be used, to allow neurological assessment. Further treatment would depend on the patient's response to current therapy.

The family would be informed that the outlook was guarded and there was still a significant probability that he would die. All we would be able to do is provide the appropriate conditions for him to get better. We would provide all treatment possible at the moment and continuously review the situation. If it became clear that he was not responding to treatment or indeed was deteriorating, we would tell the patient's family and discuss treatment withdrawal. Treatment withdrawal is a medical decision made by a group of doctors and nurses. We do not ask a patient's relatives to make these decisions; we merely want them to understand and agree with our decision.

If I had unlimited resources, the changes I would make would not be in the care that I offered to the patient, because I do not feel limited by resources in the care I can and do offer to an individual patient. However, on occasion when my unit is full, it becomes necessary to transfer a patient to another ICU or to upgrade another area and "knit" a nurse to care for the patient in that area. I would rather this were not necessary. I would want to make organizational changes so that hospitals that are able only to initially resuscitate patients like Patient A before transfer would either not provide critical care at all, transferring such patients to a regional retrieval team, or be upgraded so that appropriately trained and motivated people provide the care. If there are sufficient admissions of critically ill patients to justify this level of expenditure and maintain the skills level of the people providing the care, the unit should be upgraded. Otherwise, patients should be transferred to an appropriate facility. Sweeping up a disaster like this patient is not good medicine.

To proceed with this reorganization, information on case mix–adjusted outcome, throughput, and the number and quality of transfers, as well as information on units and hospitals, would be necessary. The purchase of intensive care treatment should be at a health authority or regional level, not at the hospital level. The provision of other services such as vascular surgery, transplantation, and upper gastrointestinal surgery would need to be considered in the distribution of units. In the United Kingdom, there are already moves within the cancer networks and, recently, the area of critical care to address these issues. The intention is to produce a managed network of services with common standards and protocols.

Patient B

According to the Department of Health,[2] patients should be admitted only if they can benefit from the care offered. The best we could return Patient B to is continuing oxygen dependence, and he would probably have new dependence on renal dialysis. His dementia would remain. Even if he were to receive critical care and survive this episode, it is very unlikely he would be accepted for long-term dialysis. One of the basic tenets of ethics is to do no harm. Admission to an ICU would prolong this man's dying but not his life. It is exceedingly unlikely that Patient B would get near an ICU in the United Kingdom; he would more likely be filtered out by the admitting medical team, who would not even discuss intensive care as an option. He would receive standard medical care on the ward. Discussion with the family would likely revolve around a do-not-resuscitate order.

It is my feeling that intensive care for Patient B would be cruel and inhumane treatment. The concept of "everything must be done" is quite unusual in the United Kingdom. I would expect discussions with the family along the lines that the kindest thing to do is to provide treatment on the ward and if he fails to respond, to allow him to die.

Assuming the worst-case scenario—that is, an accident and emergency doctor in misguided enthusiasm does indeed ventilate Patient B (relatively unlikely in the United Kingdom, because in this situation it is usual to call an intensivist or anesthetist)—the patient would only be worse at the end of a period in intensive care. There are three options available in our current protocol: 1) a do-not-resuscitate order, 2) no escalation of treatment (e.g., no inotropes, no continuous venovenous hemofiltration), and 3) treatment withdrawal.

The family members would be invited in and the options presented to them, with our chosen preference of treatment withdrawal explained. We would say, "We cannot prolong his life, only his dying. What we are currently doing to him is cruel and we should stop." I would explain that this decision had been reached by discussion and review of the patient by more than one intensivist (commonly four intensivists) plus the parent team. I would seek the family's agreement to this decision. If the relatives still insisted on continuation of care, I would try to find out why they were doing so and explain the situation, taking into account their worries. If necessary, I would bring along the renal physician to explain why he or she would not approve dialysis for this man (whose probability of 6-month survival is nil). Eventually this man will die, and it is to be hoped that death will occur sooner rather than later. Even if I won the lottery and could retire, I would not alter the management of this patient.

Patient C

In the United Kingdom, Patient C would not be offered intensive care, ventilation, and other aggressive care unless it was thought that he had a reversible condition. He has documented end-stage acquired immuno-deficiency syndrome (AIDS). He is malnourished with a chronically poisoned liver. I presume that his bleeding is from varices, though it could be from gastric or duodenal ulceration, which occurs in alcoholism. Despite his lack of muscle bulk, he has a serum creatinine level over 1000 μmol/L, which is too high for acute prerenal failure secondary to hemorrhage and indicates established renal failure. Despite having a significant hemorrhage and a hemoglobin level of 4 g/dL, he is coping well cardiovascularly.

A bleeding patient with hepatic impairment and without renal failure may respond positively if bleeding is promptly controlled. However, the combination of renal and hepatic failure is universally fatal without transplantation, which is out of the question in this case. Despite his deranged liver function, he is not yet encephalopathic and can hold a conversation; his renal failure may have a different etiology. His general debility could be related to either self-abuse and malnutrition or AIDS.

I doubt I would be asked to see this man; the parent team would almost certainly have decided that intensive care is inappropriate. If they did call me, it would be because they were not sure of the diagnoses. In this situation, I might provide baseline care and fluids, including blood, while I gathered further information. A patient with end-stage AIDS, a body mass index of 12, and renal, respiratory, and hepatic failure will not recover. After discussions with colleagues in intensive care and renal and hepatic medicine, we would discontinue active treatment and allow him to die.

I do not feel resource limited. However, it may be that my training simply leads me to unconsciously ration the care I provide. I would prefer to view my approach as providing sensible, patient-sensitive treatment. I do confess to thinking several times about how to treat this patient and to feeling a bit guilty about spending money probably pointlessly; however, I must balance this with the guilt I would feel with regard to not resuscitating a patient when the story is not entirely clear-cut and sorted in my mind.

References

[1]Hamel MB, Goldman L, Teno J, et al: Identification of comatose patients at high risk for death or severe disability. SUPPORT Investigators. Understand Prognoses and Preferences for Outcomes and Risks of Treatments. JAMA 1995;273:1842–8.

[2]Department of Health, NHS Executive: Guidelines on Admission to and Discharge From Intensive Care and High Dependency Units. London, England: Department of Health, 1996.

India

Farhad Kapadia, MD

India is a land of more than 1 billion people. That is more than the combined populations of the countries of all the other authors. Obviously, my view is only one in what is a very heterogeneous and culturally diverse country.

In our hospital, medical care is rarely if ever withheld for lack of funds. The general philosophy is that if physicians believe that therapy will be helpful, they should offer it, and it is up to management to balance the books. Thus, because I currently have relative freedom to practice medicine regardless of cost, I have only one response per patient. We do not have a running transplantation program, so I suppose if funds were unlimited, appropriate patients could be shifted abroad to the appropriate center for transplantations. Alternatively, if funds were unlimited, I suppose we could keep patients alive as long as was feasible, as an academic exercise—seeing whether any clues could be obtained, and trying any novel or experimental therapies for intractable multiple organ failure or other physiological states.

Patient A

Many questions regarding Patient A need to be answered before management is begun. One, why does a center with cardiac catheter facilities (and presumably, cardiac surgical and cardiac intensive care facilities) need to transfer such a patient? This sounds like an attempted "dump." In our setup, simply transferring the patient would not have been possible. An intensive care unit (ICU) bed would have needed to be booked before transfer of the patient, because our unit is invariably full and would not have accommodated such a patient without prior notice. Two, why was this patient transferred with a blood pressure of 78/25 mm Hg and without any inotrope or vasopressor support? Three, is there preexisting renal failure? It is unusual for a previously normal serum creatinine level to increase to 6.1 mg/dL (539 µmol/L) in 3 days. Four, after the problems during cardiac catheterization, was the infarct-related artery actually opened? Five, why is the patient not conscious? Usually, witnessed cardiac events that are followed by appropriate and successful cardiopulmonary resuscitation (CPR) do not result in significant brain damage. In fact, most patients who experience such events in the cardiac catheter room recover consciousness there. The patient's unconscious state makes one question the efficacy of the advanced cardiac life support. Was the patient conscious at *any* time after CPR? If so, that would imply that the current neurological status is due at least in part to drugs or to brain injury secondary to hypoxemia, hypotension, sepsis, and deranged metabolic parameters. Six, why is an anuric patient with a disastrous PaO_2/FIO_2 ratio still receiving intravenous fluids? Seven, why is a person who has been labeled as having sepsis not receiving antibiotics? All this makes me wonder if an intensivist was actually involved in the patient's care or if this patient was managed solely by a cardiologist. This apparent lack of early intensivist involvement meant 3 days of lost opportunities.

What would I do on arrival of the patient to the ICU? First I would decide if there was a realistic chance of brain recovery. Presuming that to be the case, I would proceed to manage the etiological events as well as correct the deranged physiology. I would have to decide whether I was dealing primarily with a cardiogenic shock state and multiple organ failure or with multiple organ failure and a septic state secondary to aspiration and acute respiratory distress syndrome. In the first hour, all initial blood tests would be performed, arterial blood gas measurements would be conducted, and a baseline electrocardiogram and a radiograph (after line insertion) would be obtained. If the primary problem was cardiogenic, there would be little to do at this stage to correct it. If it was septic, I would send off a culture screen and give the first dose of a third-generation cephalosporin.

With regard to circulatory support, I would insert an arterial and central venous line if one was not already present. (I would use a multilumen venous catheter in which the central lumen doubles up as a sheath for a pacemaker or pulmonary artery catheter, in case one should be required later.) Presuming there was no room for volume, I would start administering inotropes and vasopressors right away and get the mean arterial pressure up to at least 70 mm Hg. Simultaneously, I would request urgent echocardiography to determine if the problem is primarily cardiac, septic, or both. If the echocardiograph showed good contractility of the left ventricle and relatively low or normal estimated pulmonary artery wedge pressure, I would consider floating in a pulmonary artery catheter to help guide fluid management. If it was a clear cardiogenic picture (low left ventricular ejection fraction, high pulmonary artery wedge pressure, and low cardiac output), I would give the pulmonary artery catheter a miss. The echocardiogram would also help exclude other correctable problems, such as a pericardial collection. For the repeated premature ventricular contractions, I would obtain potassium and magnesium level measurements and start the appropriate correction. I would also consider the use of amiodarone if I thought that part of the hemodynamic instability was due to the dysrhythmia.

The patient's current arterial oxygen saturation (SaO_2) is unacceptable. I would check the baseline arterial blood gas measurements, switch to pressure control ventilation, and increase positive end-expiratory pressure to as high as hemodynamics allow. If necessary, the inspiration/expiration ratio would be inverted. I would consider it imperative to somehow get the SaO_2 above 90%, given the brain injury. If I thought that the main cause of the hypoxemia was pulmonary edema, I would consider instituting renal measures to establish diuresis. Given the cerebral status, permissive hypercapnia is not really an option. If a unilateral lung problem were predominant, I would put the patient in the lateral position with the good lung down. I would ensure that all aggressive infection prevention measures were instituted at this primary stabilization phase itself.

On the first day, after the initial first-hour resuscitation, I might insert an intra-aortic balloon pump if the circulation was not stabilized with vasopressors.

With regard to renal support, I would use standard measures to correct hyperkalemia if present. If there was a marked metabolic acidosis and a poor response to inotropes, I would partially correct the serum HCO_3 with intravenous bicarbonate. Once the inotropes had produced a reasonable mean arterial pressure, I would start furosemide with a 100-mg bolus and a drip at 40 mg/h. Renal replacement therapy would have to be started if the treatment just mentioned was clearly not working. If there was a degree of stabilization, I would consider starting some sort of enteral nutrition, preferably immunonutrition.

Later management would depend on how things were evolving. If everything was stabilizing and the patient clearly recovered consciousness, I would continue all aggressive support, and when the patient showed enough recovery, I would wean him from the support. If all systems improved but the patient showed no signs of recovering consciousness, I would give his family a realistic picture and wean him from ventilation when appropriate. He might require a tracheostomy. If he clearly recovered consciousness but remained in multiple organ failure, I would go all out with organ system support. If the primary problem was cardiogenic, I would consider another attempt to open the infarct-related artery in the catheterization laboratory.

Management would not be particularly different if I had unlimited funds. I do not have any experience with left ventricular assist devices, but I would ask more experienced colleagues if these should play any role in this case. I would also ask more experienced people if he were a candidate for cardiac transplantation.

Patient B

Patient B's case is not particularly unusual.

In our setup, we have an emergency ICU in the casualty area. Patients admitted here are not assured of transfer to the main ICU. They can be kept in this emergency ICU for a maximum of 24 hours. If not transferred to the main ICU, they then must make arrangements to transfer to another institution. If they refuse, we have the right to transfer them to a public hospital. We have not yet had to transfer patients to a public hospital, because all patients are either transferred to our ICU or to another one of the relatives' choosing. Patient B would invariably have been transferred from the emergency ICU to another institution; it is unlikely that we would have admitted this patient.

However, if we had to admit such a patient—perhaps the family is well connected or the case is a politically sensitive one—the hospital would have to bear the costs. This would be shown as charity; we have monthly and yearly targets of charity to be met.

What we would do would depend on how clearly we the physicians were communicating with the family. With rare exceptions, families are realistic and do not expect miracles or unreasonable or futile treatment. We would change the focus to ensure the comfort of the patient and his family. We would try to support the family with the help of our social worker and would allow the family relatively unlimited access to the patient's bedside.

In rare cases, the family might insist that we do everything. I often view this as a failure of communication on my part (or on the part of the whole medical community). Not infrequently, the situation is that the patient, an elderly individual, has family in a wealthier part of the world, usually the United States, and because of cultural differences or maybe guilt, the family wants everything done. We would offer standard intensive care with monitoring, administration of inotropes, and ventilation. We would use appropriate antibiotics, consider bedside desloughing of the decubital ulcers, administer artificial nutrition, and so on. If the blood pressure decreased, we would maintain an unspoken limit on the dose of inotropes. We would inform the family that the patient was sinking fast and there was nothing more we could do. No matter how insistent the relatives were, we would draw the line at renal replacement therapy or CPR—even if they threatened us with dire consequences or litigation. When the patient died, we would request corneal donation, in keeping with our "required request" policy. No cases that would guide us in these situations have yet gone through court.

In the unlikely event that the patient did actually recover, with a stable circulation and spontaneous ventilation, we would extubate him and transfer him out of the ICU. Often by this stage, the family sees the futility of this kind of management and allows the patient to receive all further therapy outside the ICU. Even if we had unlimited funds, I cannot see myself doing anything differently.

Patient C

With regard to Patient C, I have never faced a situation like this before. The following is what I think I would do: First I would inform the primary consultant that the patient was clearly not a candidate for management in the ICU. If we both agreed about this, we would tell the patient that there was nothing appropriate we could do. If I were the primary consultant, I would tell him the same thing. Usually, regardless who the primary consultant is, I speak directly to the family about the possible outcomes of intensive care. Also, normally under these circumstances, we do not spell out the options of intubation, ventilation, renal replacement therapy, and so on. Considering that the options had already been mentioned and the patient was demanding them all, I would inform him that we could not accommodate him in our ICU but that we could transport him to a public hospital.

If, on the other hand, the primary consultant insisted that we do everything, I would initiate a quick and focused discussion about filling beds in our ICU with patients being given futile treatment, and I would inform him or her that this attitude, if also taken up by other consultants, would result in a filled ICU, with no physicians getting beds for sick patients who would respond to salvage treatment, and with elective work being needlessly canceled. If the primary consultant still insisted, I suppose I would admit the patient, insert the appropriate lines, stabilize the circulation, correct the coagulopathy, start administering appropriate antimicrobials, and use noninvasive ventilation. Unless tremendous pressure was placed on me, I would not intubate and ventilate this patient. Similarly, I would not ask my nephrology colleagues to begin hemodialysis; they would have concurred with my decision not to use renal replacement therapy. In our given socioeconomic climate, it is unlikely that we can be forced into offering futile therapy.

What if I were a physician in a public hospital and had no choice except to admit the patient? I still believe that I would follow the same course (that is, admit, ensure basic medical care, but not offer aggressive intensive care involving intubation, ventilation, or renal replacement therapy). Given the lack of funds, I do not see authorities questioning this line of action.

If I had unlimited funds, beds, and staff, I suppose I would try everything, more with hope than with conviction. About a decade ago, we were pessimistic about saving the lives of acquired immunodeficiency syndrome (AIDS) patients who had *Pneumocystis carinii* pneumonia and who required ventilation. We thought this was an inappropriate use of ICU beds. Now we can save the lives of a large number of these patients.

In a similar vein, I would reason that if we could get this patient through this crisis, given the rapid advances in AIDS medicine we might possibly address the immediate future of AIDS treatment (e.g., antiretroviral therapy, intense counseling, home support). After all, he is only 42 years old. At present, however, advanced holistic treatment for patients with AIDS is only a fantasy in India.

New Zealand

Stephen Streat, MD

Patient A

Before I comment on Patient A's case, let me make three observations.

First, in New Zealand there are no cardiac care units to which intubated patients can go. Ventilatory support is provided only in the emergency department (ED), operating room, and intensive care unit (ICU). Patients in coronary care units who require intubation in an emergency are ventilated by hand for a few minutes and are then assessed by intensivists, who will take them to the ICU should intermittent positive-pressure ventilation and other intensive therapies be thought appropriate.

Second, intensive care in New Zealand is not provided by cardiologists or other "single organ doctors." It is the responsibility of intensivists. Intensive care medicine is recognized as a separate specialty by the Medical Council of New Zealand.[1]

Third, no one in New Zealand is transferred for continuing care to an ICU without the prior agreement of the intensivist responsible for that ICU.

For the sake of argument then, I will assume that the patient has been referred to me from "St. Elsewhere's" ICU, where the standard of care was less than what I would ordinarily expect when referred a patient such as this.

Patient A is a 57-year-old man with severe multiple organ failure, including hypoxic-ischemic encephalopathy (HIE) of possibly severe extent (compounded by sedation and renal failure). He has persistent shock, acute respiratory distress syndrome (ARDS), and severe renal failure. The extent of the multiple organ failure is consistent with being around 5 days post-arrest. This patient would be admitted to ICU for assessment only if the degree to which his encephalopathy was compounded by residual sedation could not be determined by taking a careful history. Given the apparently inadequate standard of care that he has received (e.g., no vasopressors, untreated hypoxia and hypotension, inappropriate fluid therapy), it seems unlikely that a reliable history of sedation could be obtained.

Under such circumstances, we might admit the patient to the ICU to determine the neurological prognosis and provide supportive care until that determination could be made. This type of admission is known as an admission with reservations. It represents the first level of three stages of limitation of intensive therapies (reservations, specific limitations, and withdrawal are the three stages) that are an integral part of the way we practice. Admitting a patient with reservations acts as a signal that intensive therapies may be limited or withdrawn if the patient does not make good progress. In this situation, intensive therapies (including, for example, correction of hypoxia, correction of hypotension, and clearing of residual sedation by dialysis) might be administered for 48 hours, pending an assessment of neurological status and reversibility of multiple organ failure. The assessment might include various neurological tests (magnetic resonance imaging, electroencephalography, somatosensory evoked potential testing) in addition to serial neurological examinations. Should this assessment show that severe HIE was present, intensive therapies would be withdrawn by the intensivists in the context of consensus among any other treating physicians and the patient's family.

Alternatively, if it was clear (for example, on visiting the ICU of referral and examining the patient and his clinical record) that the central nervous system situation at the time of referral to our ICU was not compounded by sedation, I would decline to admit this patient to our ICU and would write a note such as this in the clinical record:

> Thank you for asking me to see this 57-year-old man with severe multiple organ failure. He is now 5 days post–cardiopulmonary resuscitation (CPR), following cardiac arrest during angioplasty at the time of acute inferior infarction. Currently, he is in poor condition. He has had no sedation for 48 hours and has received intermittent low-dose opioid only for the previous 48 hours. No limb response to deep pain has ever been documented post-CPR. He currently grimaces to deep pain but has no eye-opening or limb response to deep pain. He has no lash reflex but has intact corneal and oculocephalic reflexes and reactive pupils. These findings were unaltered by administration of 0.8 mg of intravenous naloxone. He has severe ARDS, secondary to aspiration, and is still in shock, with established anuric renal failure. It appears that hypovolemia has not been corrected, but he has poor cardiac function, documented by echocardiography (inferior and septal akinesis, ejection fraction 32%) and pulmonary artery catheter monitoring (cardiac index 2.5, despite pulmonary artery wedge pressure of 19 mm Hg) during the first few days postarrest. In my opinion, further intensive therapies are inappropriate, given the patient's severe HIE. Accordingly, admission to the Department of Critical Care Medicine is declined.

I have discussed this case with several of my intensivist colleagues and we are all in agreement. The patient's severe multiple organ failure is multifactorial, including aspiration and cardiogenic shock post-CPR, and he may now have early nosocomial pneumonia. This syndrome alone would carry a high mortality, especially in the absence of mechanically reversible cardiac dysfunction. I suggest that you discuss this situation fully and frankly with the patient's family and advise the family that intensive therapies be withdrawn and a comfort care plan be instituted. We would be happy to give further advice on request.

Although we are limited to 14 beds capable of supporting mechanical ventilation, we are able in emergency situations to take more patients, and we would not deny a clinically suitable and appropriate patient admission solely on the grounds of resource constraint.[2] We have at our disposal a full range of intensive therapies and supportive services, in keeping with the Australian and New Zealand standard for an academic tertiary-level ICU.[3]

Patient B

As with the first case, there are important differences in the way in which Patient B would be treated before referral to an ICU in New Zealand.

First, the patient would not be intubated and given mechanical ventilation because the relatives wanted everything done. We intensivists would not do this, and the emergency medicine specialists would not do it either. If by some remote chance a foreign visiting emergency physician did it, the story would probably be on national television, presented like this: "Crazy doctors torture frail old man in bizarre technological imperative, while poor John Victim has been waiting in pain for his angioplasty for the last 3 months."

Second, the patient would not be transferred to our medical ICU. In New Zealand, ICUs are "closed" and are accessed only with the prior knowledge and consent of the intensivist and in accord with written admission and discharge policies (see, for example, the article by Streat and Judson[2]). I, and all of my colleagues, would certainly deny this patient admission—irrespective of the expressed wishes of the patient, his family, or any referring physician or of the amount of intensive care resources available at the time. Furthermore, we would never wish intensive care resources to be so great that the admission of patients like Patient B was expected by our society. Should such a situation develop, we would advocate that those resources be used in other areas of health care.

Patient B is an 88-year-old man with severe sepsis, possibly from a pulmonary source—perhaps postaspiration. He has diabetes, hypertension, peripheral vascular disease, atherosclerotic heart disease, chronic renal insufficiency, chronic hypoxic respiratory failure, and dementia. He lives in a skilled nursing home but has decubiti and cachexia and cannot perform self-care. In association with sepsis, he has developed worsening hypoxia, shock, anuric renal failure, and coma. This syndrome is not reversible, except by virtue of astronomically unlikely good fortune, considerable time in the ICU, and great expense. Even if it were reversible, he would at best be a very old man dying slowly from chronic multiple organ failure.

If I consulted on this patient in the ED (which is extremely unlikely and has never occurred in my career to date), I would say:

> Thank you for asking me to consider for ICU admission this 88-year-old man with multiple comorbidities, including cachexia, dementia, and chronic renal and respiratory failure. He has a poor level of daily functioning; he receives 24-hour nursing care and is unable to perform self-care. He presents now with septic shock from infected pressure areas or from a pulmonary etiology and with severe multiple organ failure. He was intubated and ventilated by a locum specialist emergency physician before consultation with physicians in the ICU. In my opinion and that of three of my colleagues, continuation of intensive therapies is inappropriate in this case. We suggest that you explain this to the patient's family and reach an agreement with the family that that these be withdrawn. We would be happy to assist with this process on your request.

I would also ask the clinical director of the ED to subject the case to internal medical audit in that department and to inform me of the result of the audit.

Patient C

As with the first two cases, Patient C's case is simply unrealistic in New Zealand. Given that the patient has unremitting alcoholism and is not compliant with antiretroviral therapy, it is likely that these medications would have already been withdrawn by his infectious disease physicians. Further, with regard to the statement "When options are read to him, he desires them all," no "options" would be read to him. In New Zealand, intensive care is not offered à la carte, with patients choosing to partake in whole or in part—it is more a "package deal by invitation only."

Patient C is a 42-year-old man with extensive ethanol dependency and acquired immunodeficiency syndrome (AIDS) who has continued to drink heavily despite medical advice, has repeatedly declined rehabilitation, and is noncompliant with his antiretroviral therapy. He presents with cachexia, jaundice, and massive upper gastrointestinal bleeding, and he has probably aspirated. Laboratory results show severe renal failure and hepatic derangement with marked coagulopathy. The platelet count is not listed but is likely very low, given his alcohol use, folate deficiency, hepatic failure, massive bleeding, and pathologic oozing; the antiretrovirals may also play a role. This is likely due to alcoholic cirrhosis, variceal bleeding, and, possibly, opportunistic infection.

The underlying diseases (alcoholism and AIDS) are neither reversible nor controllable in this noncompliant patient. Further, the patient's physiological deterioration is severe, and the probability of reversing that derangement, even with aggressive intensive therapies, is very low. Even if by some miracle the patient survived, he would still be a noncompliant man with cachexia, AIDS, and alcoholism. This patient would therefore not meet our written admission criteria[2] and would be declined admission.

If I were called to see him in the ED, I would not intubate and ventilate him but would immediately call my hepatology and infectious disease colleagues (who at some time would have prescribed his antiretrovirals) and arrive at a consensus plan that would not involve the use of intensive therapies.

I would then tell the patient, "You are bleeding very fast from what we think are ruptured high-pressure veins in the gullet. These are due to cirrhosis of the liver. Your blood does not clot because of your liver disease, and so we can't stop this bleeding. Your breathing is difficult because you have breathed some of the vomited blood into your lungs. Your kidneys have stopped working, and it looks as if this occurred quite some time ago. I'm afraid that we cannot fix these problems. I'm sorry. We will take care of you and look after you, but these are very serious problems and I'm afraid that you might die. We can give you some medication to help with your breathing and your vomiting. Do you have any family members or friends we can call to come and be with you?"

A note with similar content would be written for the medical record. This approach to the patient would be the same regardless of the amount of resources available for intensive care.

This is an emotionally charged situation, full of sound and color, especially in an ED resuscitation room, and I would therefore seek to transfer the patient to a low-technology environment outside the ED or the ICU. My colleagues in infectious disease or hepatology would oblige and take over the management of this patient.

References

[1]Medical Council of New Zealand: Professional standards. Available at: http://www.mcnz.org.nz/standards. Accessed November 11, 2001.

[2]Streat S, Judson JA: Cost containment: the Pacific. New Zealand. New Horiz 1994;2:392–403.

[3]Faculty of Intensive Care, Australian and New Zealand College of Anaesthetists: Policy documents. Available at: http://www.fic.anzca.edu.au/policy/index.htm. Accessed November 11, 2001.

The Netherlands

Hans van der Spoel, MD

When doctors in the Netherlands, like probably all over the world, graduate from medical school, they take an oath—the Hippocratic Oath. They vow that they will treat every patient who seeks their help, respect the patient, act in his or her best interests, and first of all do no harm. This situation is according to our laws and confirmed in numerous court decisions. This attitude toward treatment also implies that medically futile treatment should be avoided, because this is not in the patient's best interest. Doctors must withhold inappropriate treatment and stop treatment that is no longer appropriate. This was underscored in the following two cases, taken to court in the Netherlands:

A premature newborn with congenital cerebral, cardiac, and digestive tract defects was expected to survive for only a short period. Shortly after birth, before further investigations could be done, the infant was intubated and ventilated. One of the defects was esophageal atresia. The doctors did not consider it appropriate to operate for this, because operating would only prolong the suffering of this infant, who was expected to die within a couple of weeks. The parents, however, wanted everything done. Many discussions between doctors and parents followed, in which the medical side was explained over and over. The parents persisted in their view, and ultimately they went to court to force the surgeons to operate. The judge recognized the medical autonomy in this case, arguing that it was up to the medical experts to determine whether an operation would be medically futile. The child was not operated on and died shortly after.

The second case is that of an 88-year-old man in a bad general condition after multiple cerebral infarctions. He was operated on for an obstructing carcinoma of the colon. The tumor could not be removed completely, and hepatic metastases were found as well. Some days after the operation, the patient needed respiratory support because of pneumonia. Although the operating surgeon had stated that no heroic measures were to be undertaken (i.e., no resuscitation and no intensive care), these restrictions had not been entered into the medical chart. Of course, it was the middle of the night when the patient came to the hospital in need of respiratory support, and he was admitted to the intensive care unit (ICU), intubated, and so on. In a discussion the next day with the patient's only daughter, the intensivists said that the admission to the ICU should not have occurred, given the limited prognosis. Now that he had been admitted, however, he would be treated in such a way that he could be extubated after the pulmonary problems had resolved, but new major complications would not be treated.

The daughter was furious and demanded that everything be done. During his prolonged stay in the ICU, these items were discussed repeatedly by the medical staff and the daughter, without any change in points of view. At last the patient was extubated and discharged to a step-down unit, but it was decided that he was not to come back to the ICU. The daughter went to court, requesting that her father be admitted to the ICU if he needed respiratory support again. The doctors stated that given this man's advanced carcinoma and very bad general condition, a new admission would be senseless and would only prolong a situation of medical futility—he was expected to die within a couple of weeks. The court ruled that it was up to the physicians to judge whether a medical treatment was justified or futile and that a new admission to the ICU could not be forced if the doctors thought it useless.

So doctors in the Netherlands are granted the right to decide whether medical treatment is justified or not. Patients, legal representatives, and family are basically excluded from this decision-making process, although their opinions are to be heard. Of course, patients have the right to refuse treatment they do not want to undergo, but they cannot claim treatment.

None of the three patients whose cases are discussed in this book have health insurance. In the Netherlands, however, virtually everyone has health insurance, which covers almost everything except really "luxury" medical treatment (e.g., cosmetic surgery). Physicians are obliged to treat (and hospitals to pay for the treatment of) every patient who is in acute need of medical care, no matter whether the illness is life threatening or potentially disabling or may lead to a worse medical condition. If a patient does not have health insurance, the hospital gets most of the money back from the social insurance, which in turn tries to get the money from the patient, although in fact this is seldom accomplished. In the same way, uninsured patients from abroad are offered necessary medical treatment. Many countries have bilateral treaties covering financial compensation for medical services offered to their citizens traveling abroad. So whether a patient has health insurance is irrelevant in treating serious conditions.

In addition, Dutch physicians—at least physicians in our ICU—are permitted to administer without serious financial restrictions nearly any available medical treatment. Only new, experimental therapies are discussed with hospital administration. No differences are made between rich or "valuable" individuals and poor, homeless, human immunodeficiency virus (HIV)-positive, or drug-addicted persons or illegal aliens.

Patient A

It would be tricky to get Patient A transferred, because he might be beyond cerebral repair, but no good evaluation can be made at this stage, given his condition. Even if grimacing were considered to imply a motor score of 5, a Glasgow Coma Scale score of less than 8 on day 3 postresuscitation is indicative of at least serious brain damage. Normal procedure in our department in cases of coma due to anoxic brain damage is as follows: Test somatosensory evoked potentials on day 3. If there are no somatosensory evoked N20 potentials via either the left or right nervus medianus, stop further therapy, because prognosis for cerebral recovery is poor. If somatosensory evoked potentials are not absent but electroencephalography indicates serious damage, gradually withdraw therapy, depending on overall neurological examination findings and prognosis regarding cardiac function. Regardless of the findings, we would likely make an effort in the case of this seriously undertreated patient, referred from another hospital.

First I would optimize circulation. Goals would be a cardiac index greater than 3 and a mean arterial pressure greater than 70 mm Hg (to optimize cerebral perfusion pressure, because of postanoxia brain damage; in normal brains, a mean arterial pressure greater than 60 mm Hg would do).

I would make an assessment using transesophageal echocardiography in combination with a more objective method of measuring cardiac output (Swan-Ganz catheter monitoring, CO_2-rebreathing cardiac output measurement, esophageal Doppler ultrasonography, or a combination). Vasoactive medication would include dopamine, ketanserin (and/or nitroglycerin), enoximone (or another phosphodiesterase inhibitor), and norepinephrine (if needed to maintain arterial pressure). Fluid resuscitation would be guided clinically or by one or more of the aforementioned techniques for measuring cardiac output. I might insert an intra-aortic balloon pump, depending if there was any ongoing infarction and/or myocardial ischemia. I would give magnesium for premature ventricular contractions and add amiodarone if they persisted. I would improve (micro)circulation by augmenting cardiac output. Use of vasodilators would take care of the hypoxic damage to liver and pancreas and would prevent ischemic ("stress") ulcers. If the knees are warm, the patient is in good circulatory condition.

Second, I would optimize ventilation or oxygenation. Methods would include prone positioning, positive end-expiratory pressure as needed, pressure control ventilation, and recruitment maneuvers. I would keep PCO_2 at about 40 mm Hg (no permissive hypercapnia would be used to promote cerebral vasodilation in this case). I guess that within 3 hours, FIO_2 could be reduced to 40%.

Third, I would increase diuresis and start renal replacement therapy. Furosemide 1250 mg/24 h would be started via continuous infusion for 5 hours. I would stop this treatment if urine output did not increase significantly. Continuous venovenous hemofiltration would be considered; it is our experience that this improves circulation and cardiac function.

Fourth, I would treat the inflammation and infection and prevent new infections. I would give dexamethasone 1 mg/kg followed by a tapering course of prednisolone; this would reduce the hyperinflammatory response and capillary leakage, increase renal perfusion, and augment receptor sensitivity to catecholamines. I would give cefotaxime and ciprofloxacin with selective decontamination of the digestive tract (SDD), after obtaining samples for culture (blood, sputum, throat, and feces/rectum). I would adjust or stop antibiotics after preliminary culture results arrived. I would start with broad-spectrum antibiotics because I do not know the microbial environment of the referring hospital. Selective decontamination of the digestive tract would virtually eliminate further secondary endogenous infections. New central lines would be placed; I never trust lines placed in another hospital.

Fifth, the head of the bed would be elevated to 30 degrees to improve venous return from the head; this might also reduce intracranial pressure somewhat.

Sixth, I would measure antithrombin III levels and other parameters to check for diffuse intravascular coagulation, and I would correct any coagulation deficiencies.

Seventh, I would start enteral feeding, which would include administration of glutamine, arginine, and ω-3 fatty acids.

Eighth, I would tell the family that the prognosis was grim, especially in terms of cerebral function. I would explain that we were trying to improve the patient's general condition and that maybe with optimizing of his general function, his cerebral function would improve. If, however, his cerebral condition were not to improve, and especially if somatosensory evoked potentials were absent, all therapy would be stopped, because he would never regain consciousness.

Finally, I would contact the referring hospital and would tell the administrators to stop intervention cardiology if they did not improve their intensive care. I would consider informing the health authorities.

Patient B

The chances that Patient B will survive his period in the ICU, even if everything is done, are very, very small. The Acute Physiology and Chronic Health Evaluation II–predicted mortality would be something like 90%, even without consideration of his cachexia and his dependency on others for help with activities of daily living. Even if he were to survive his stay in the ICU, his physiological reserves are so small that he would surely develop a new, probably lethal, complication while on the ward. All in all, there are no realistic chances that intensive care would do him any good; it would only postpone death. He would not be admitted to our ICU. Apart from the fact that almost no doctor in our hospital would even consider admitting this patient to the ICU, we have a "closed" ICU, so no patient enters without being evaluated by one of our staff. If Patient B was intubated by paramedics while being transported from his nursing home to our emergency department (ED), we would keep him in the ED, explain the situation to his relatives, give them some time, and extubate him. If he did not die shortly after extubation, he would be admitted to the general ward for palliative care.

Patient C

Patient C has severe acute-on-chronic (at least liver, and probably brain) multiple organ failure, with active gastrointestinal bleeding and chronic liver disease along with complications affecting coagulation and his respiratory, hepatic, renal, circulatory, gastrointestinal, and central nervous systems. His white blood cell count of 34,000/mm^3 seems to indicate that his HIV infection is not very advanced, but an opportunistic infection or a malignancy cannot be excluded at this stage. Leukocytosis may be due to a nonopportunistic infection (spontaneous bacterial peritonitis?), pneumonia, or stress. Regarding the HIV infection, his prognosis might be rather good— if he were compliant with therapy. The same holds true for his liver disease, assuming he stopped drinking alcohol. Liver transplantation is not indicated, given his HIV infection.

If the emergency doctor phoned me about this patient, I would probably not even go to see the patient myself. I would simply say that we could do nothing for him. If, however, somebody such as his family doctor convinced me that the patient was waiting for just such an event (this bleeding episode) to become a compliant, abstinent patient, I might give him a chance, in part because this would be a good training case for fellows on the staff. That is, we might admit him and treat him for a few days. If we could get him in a better condition with improving parameters and stop the upper gastrointestinal bleeding, we would go on. If, however, therapy was not successful (further deterioration of his coagulation, increasing serum ammonia level, rebleeding), we would discontinue therapy after a maximum of 3–4 days.

This scenario is very unlikely and is independent of the patient's desires. Admission to the ICU is the doctor's decision. In the unlikely event that we admitted him, we would intubate and ventilate him, give him packed red blood cells and plasma, perform upper gastrointestinal tract endoscopy with band ligation of his varices or sclerotherapy for his gastric bleeding (if bleeding could not be stopped, we would then stop all therapy right then), start intravenous octreotide therapy, start continuous venovenous hemofiltration, administer laxatives and neostigmine to promote cleansing of the bowels, and initiate SDD and a short course of cefotaxime (after ascites culture). We would give him every vitamin we had available, especially thiamine. If he survived and was discharged from the hospital and had even one more alcoholic drink, I would never admit the patient again. However, I know of some alcoholic patients, though not many, who remained abstinent after their first ICU admission.

In this case, admitting the patient is as justified as refusing admission. In our ICU, the intensivist in charge can decide what he or she wants, and everybody in the ICU would comply, but only after much discussion and with the expectation of clear improvement after a maximum of several days.

Russia

Michael Karakozov, MD

Each patient in the intensive care unit (ICU) must be admitted by one of the clinical departments according to the leading syndrome. The attending physician (usually the chief of the department), not an intensivist, develops the general treatment plan and prognosis, both of which must be documented in the chart. The intensivist on duty (me) monitors the patient's vital functions (e.g., hemodynamics, perfusion, oxygenation, diuresis) and carries out the treatment plan of the responsible attending. A big problem is that there are no standards of care in our ICU, only recommendations and sometimes guidelines. Care is largely guided by the personal experiences of the intensivist, based on the range of the hospital's resources.

Patient A

Patient A would immediately go to the ICU. The first question on admission would be, what department takes the patient—cardiology or pulmonology? Assuming a myocardial infarction was not the major reason for this patient's critical state, most probably he would have an attending pulmonologist and consulting cardiologist while receiving treatment in our ICU.

Patient A's treatment plan most likely would include the following:

Restoration of perfusion and oxygenation: I would choose a non-invasive blood pressure monitor, a central venous catheter, and a pulse oximeter. I would begin controlled mechanical ventilation with positive end-expiratory pressure (PEEP). Titration of PEEP would be done with concomitant infusions of fluid, to ensure normal or nearly normal cardiac output. If I managed to restore normal blood pressure with infusion of crystalloids without worsening of the patient's lung edema, I would steadily increase PEEP and decrease FIO_2. If not, I would switch to inotropes (I think dopamine is the most appropriate agent), but only if I took care of the tachycardia and premature ventricular contractions, should they persist after cardiac output restoration. I would want to have the patient's arterial oxygen saturation (SaO_2) greater than 90%. The ventilation mode would be changed to a less aggressive one at the earliest opportunity.

Antibiotic therapy: Antibiotic therapy would be empiric, and the attending pulmonologist would be responsible for selection. Most probably, this patient would receive a third-generation cephalosporin.

Treatment of oliguria: If oliguria persisted after fluid infusions, I would administer furosemide (up to 0.5 g). If this did not work, I would attempt short-term hemodialysis. At the moment, no continuous renal replacement therapies are available. If I could not treat oliguria conventionally, the patient's prognosis would be seriously affected.

I think that no specific therapy for inferior myocardial infarction 3 days after onset is available. This patient would receive all available medications and treatment, despite his lack of insurance.

If I had unlimited resources, this would be my treatment plan:

Restoration of perfusion and oxygenation: To monitor hemodynamics, I would insert a pulmonary artery catheter. Monitoring all pressures and assessing cardiac output would be done to guide titration of fluids and inotropes and optimal ventilatory support. I would start with lactated Ringer's and glucose-insulin-potassium solutions, to restore a nearly normal cardiac index and reduce the tachycardia. Then I would administer inotropes (most likely dopamine) and antiarrhythmics (lidocaine) if premature ventricular contractions remained frequent.

I would assess the patient's cardiac and pulmonary status on admission by echocardiography and lung computed tomography (together with chest radiography), if doing so would not interfere with the immediate treatment. I would not start with permissive hypercapnia or any other small-tidal-volume, high-PEEP ventilation techniques (hyperventilation on admission would be more appropriate) but would consider them after volume and cardiac output restoration and attenuation of ventricular arrhythmia, tachycardia, and metabolic acidosis. Frequent blood gas analyses as well as calculation of pulmonary shunt would be performed. Sodium bicarbonate would be given if there was severe acidosis. Gastric tonometry would be used to monitor regional perfusion. Electrocardiography, pulse oximetry, and capnography would be performed.

Treatment of sepsis: I would arrange analysis of blood and bronchial lavage cultures and sensitivities in order to make the best antibiotic choice. Pending the results, I would use a cephalosporin empirically. Serum antibiotic concentrations would be measured after initiation of treatment. Daily blood cell counts and serum analysis for known septic mediators would continue.

Improvement of renal function: If renal function did not improve after fluid replacement, I would consider furosemide and dopamine infusion. If furosemide therapy had no effect in the first 24 hours, I would switch to continuous renal replacement therapy such as venovenous hemodiafiltration. Strict control of fluid balance and weight monitoring would be mandatory, with electrolytes checked at least twice a day.

Treatment of coagulation disorders: Platelet levels, prothrombin time, partial thromboplastin time, and clotting factor levels (if abnormal) would be monitored daily for the first 3 days. Vitamin K would be considered, but a mild increase in prothrombin time without clinical bleeding would not be important in this patient. Sucralfate therapy would be administered as acute ulcer prophylaxis. The mode of ventilatory support would be chosen on the basis of PO_2, SaO_2, lung mechanics, and cardiac function. Modern techniques such as prone ventilation, exogenous surfactant administration, and even gene therapy (if other methods failed) could be considered to ameliorate the acute respiratory distress syndrome. I would decrease FIO_2 and give less aggressive ventilatory support as soon as possible.

Patient B

It is very unlikely that Patient B would be admitted to our ICU. There are two nursing homes here, but these patients are never admitted to our hospital. Admission would be possible, I guess, if the patient had relatives or friends who were physicians, wealthy "new Russians," or local officials. Paternalism still runs deep in people's minds, and people usually believe what the doctor says. Under the newly adopted laws in Russia, people have the right to insist on any kind of treatment that is available through the local hospital. Very few exercise their rights; the traditional communist mentality remains. Things are steadily improving, but very slowly. If a hospital cannot provide optimal treatment, consideration would be given to transferring the patient in question to another medical establishment with better facilities. Patients must have insurance or know somebody who will pay for treatment. Cash at every level accelerates the process.

So I will assume that Patient B was admitted to our hospital and ICU after a call from somebody with influence. He has multiple organ failure and has developed septic complications (most obviously acute pneumonia or urosepsis); his background dementia seriously worsens the prognosis. Knowing our facilities and level of care, I have to admit that he will inevitably die. Transportation to a center in St. Petersburg or Moscow is unlikely because we do not have equipped helicopters and the patient's unstable condition makes transportation extremely risky, if not impossible.

What would I do? First I would consult with a nephrologist, a cardiologist, and a pulmonologist, as well as with someone from the hospital administration. Second, I would have the administration talk to the patient's relatives. The paternalistic approach would serve its purpose in this situation. Even if his relatives were all wealthy medical workers sitting at the political summit, they would consider the prognosis and agree that our treatment would be futile. But they might insist on complete comfort care before the patient died. This we would provide.

If the patient had no insurance but powerful relatives who insisted on aggressive management, the hospital would have to do everything it could. I would have to call every consulting specialist to the ICU. If this patient had "ordinary" relatives, he would not receive any expensive treatment and I would be asked not to prolong his agony but rather to make it less painful for him. There would be no standards of care except one: euthanasia is strictly forbidden. What would I do? I could continue administering a first-generation cephalosporin and perform rapid venovenous ultrafiltration to ameliorate his pulmonary edema. Inotropes could then be used, with great caution not to precipitate iatrogenic arrhythmia. I would start giving intravenous insulin. There would be no chance of continuous renal replacement and only a small chance of intermittent hemodialysis. The patient would be sedated and would receive control or assist/control mode ventilation, and FIO_2 would be titrated according to his SaO_2 (targeted to more than 90% if possible). Repeated radiography would be done to monitor the pulmonary edema. There is nothing more I could do.

If I had unlimited resources, my approach to treatment would be somewhat different. The patient has a long history of chronic illness. Infection has acutely compromised his weak organ systems. Treating his acute pathology effectively means breaking the vicious cycle at many points. If untreated, these points can quickly lead to death. If they are treated effectively and the patient has enough reserve (which I strongly doubt he has), theoretically I could restore him to the condition he was in before emergency admission. Nobody can predict with 100% certainty the effect of early aggressive though costly treatment, but everybody can doubt its use. I try to follow the simple known formula in my practice: intensive care must restore the patient's vital (i.e., life) functions and not prolong dying.

Is this patient dying, or has he only a potentially treatable acute infectious process with chronic pathology? I believe that he is dying and has being slowly dying for a long time. The way I can assist nature is to make the final stage of this process as painless as possible.

The difficult ethical question for me is whether, if I had all the up-to-date technologies, laboratories, and staff, I could make the determination that death was inevitable. Should I try to treat? At least begin? I think I would, because I have never had the chance to see the results of modern expensive technologies. There is a good proverb: It is better to die according to the rules of treatment than to survive despite them. At least the patient's relatives would agree with me.

Every step would be discussed with the pulmonologist, nephrologist, endocrinologist, and cardiologist. To begin with, I would consider immediate ultrafiltration followed by continuous hemodialysis; use of strong, effective antibiotics chosen on the basis of rapidly obtained blood, urine, and sputum culture results; and correction of acidosis with bicarbonate and blood sugar levels with insulin. Conventional mechanical ventilation would be begun in control mode and be switched to a less aggressive one as soon as possible. I would try to stabilize cardiac performance and perfusion with a complex cocktail of inotropes, vasodilators, and antiarrhythmics while I quickly addressed the problem of pulmonary edema and started hemodialysis. I would perform invasive assessment of cardiac function and provide gastric ulcer prophylaxis.

I realize that all this treatment might be futile and expensive, but I would be unable to resist the temptation to try it.

Patient C

Patient C has a very poor prognosis. We have not yet seen patients with documented acquired immunodeficiency syndrome (AIDS) in our ICU and do not have any experience with *Pneumocystis carinii* pneumonia and other AIDS-related opportunistic infections. It is quite possible that some of our immunocompromised patients were not purely alcoholic or drug-abusing patients. Our diagnoses may have been as poor as their liver transaminase concentrations.

Patient C is likely to die from end-stage liver cirrhosis, hemorrhage with coagulopathy, hepatorenal syndrome, and respiratory failure. At our hospital, this would not be an unusual case, but I am not sure whether common approaches to these patients exist in different clinics in Russia or the former Soviet Union. Maybe somewhere in Moscow, Siberia, or the Far Eastern Region, someone might have thought of sending this man to the ICU from the emergency department. Time is needed to establish and maintain specific protocols for responding to different kinds of fatal and nonfatal illnesses.

Everybody knows that this patient's case is hopeless. However, there is a strong traditional rule, almost a strict law, at our hospital: the patient must not die of uncontrolled hemorrhage, no matter what the cause. This approach is quite primitive. Nevertheless, I would admit this man to the ICU and begin blood transfusions. If he had developed hepatic coma without hemorrhage, I would not have had to admit him to the ICU and he would have died on the gastroenterology or nephrology service without even a critical care consultation.

In the ICU, the attending surgeon would perform an endoscopy to find the bleeding varices and then would introduce a Blakemore tube. I would transfuse packed red blood cells and fresh frozen plasma. That would be all. Then everybody would wait until the decompensated patient died from coagulopathy, coma, respiratory failure, or multiple organ failure. If, while the patient was alive, his AIDS status was mentioned, in a second he would be without even nursing care. Sometimes there are not enough gloves for staff to work safely. If the attending surgeon documented the patient's grave prognosis, I would have the right not to intubate and to withhold all expensive medications. That is why I cannot see any sense in expensive transfusions.

If resources were unlimited, the prognosis would still be poor. I would place a nasogastric tube, sedate the man, even intubate him, and let him die peacefully. I discussed this scenario with my colleagues because I was curious to know how much effort others would devote to this patient if they were lucky to have everything at their disposal. Nobody gave him any chance of survival. The only addition they would make to what I would offer is mechanical ventilation until he died, if apnea or hypopnea developed after sedation. But they would use only a very simple, old Soviet high-frequency ventilator.

I think that in intensive care, the result of treatment is more important than the process, for why else would physicians employ numerous costly and invasive methods, with the risk of possibly fatal complications? The ultimate aim of intensive care is to support and restore failed vital functions. Even if I could support hepatic function with liver transplantation, renal function with dialysis, cardiac function with inotropes or antiarrhythmics, coagulatory function with separate transfusions of every possible factor, and respiration with mechanical ventilation or extracorporeal membrane oxygenation, what could I do in the face of an immunodeficiency that would destroy each of these functions easily and quickly? I cannot achieve and predict good outcomes on the basis of up-to-date knowledge and machinery in this case, but I can help nature to make the process of dying painless. Why not do this?

Hong Kong

Ian K.S. Tan, MBBS

Patient A

On admission of Patient A to the intensive care unit (ICU), the placement of the tracheal tube would be checked and pressure control ventilation would be begun with an inspiratory time of 50%. A central venous catheter and arterial catheter would be inserted, low-dose epinephrine (less than 8 μg/min) would be started immediately, and preload would be assessed by echocardiography and by ascertaining the systolic pressure variation and noninvasive cardiac output, among other parameters. If preload was deemed high, positive end-expiratory pressure (PEEP) would be increased to 16 cm H_2O to reduce preload and afterload and improve oxygenation. If preload was assessed to be low, fluid would be given in titrated boluses before PEEP was increased. If the blood pressure failed to improve, norepinephrine would be titrated to achieve a mean arterial pressure of at least 70 mm Hg.

On attainment of hemodynamic goals, which should occur within an hour of ICU admission, zero-balanced continuous hemodiafiltration with regional citrate anticoagulation would be started, with a prescribed urea clearance of at least 2000 mL/h. If preload was high, slow continuous ultrafiltration with dialysis would be prescribed. If oxygenation did not improve despite 100% FIO_2, PEEP, and ultrafiltration, the patient would receive inverse ratio pressure control ventilation.

In addition, arterial blood gas and phosphate level measurements would be obtained and cultures of blood, sputum, and urine would be sent. A nasogastric tube and a urinary catheter would be placed if not already in situ. A physical examination would be done. The family would be interviewed, necessary consents for treatment obtained, and information given about the patient's current status, treatment, prognosis, and management plan. Psychosocial support would be provided.

Enteral feeding would be started at 10 mL/h, to be increased every 4 hours if tolerated, according to protocol. Sucralfate would be prescribed, and if the nasogastric tube returned blood, a histamine-2-receptor blocker would be prescribed instead. The length of the patient's hospital stay was not mentioned; the first-generation cephalosporin would be continued if the pneumonia was not complicated by nosocomial organisms. Otherwise, the antibiotic regimen would be broadened to cover the probable infecting organism (if any) and its sensitivities. Intravenous infusions of morphine and midazolam would be titrated to achieve analgesia and comfort. These infusions would then be intermittently discontinued in order to assess neurological status.

The cardiologist would be asked to review the patient's case, to consider obtaining serial echocardiograms, and to discuss issues related to placement of an intra-aortic balloon pump and myocardial revascularization. The ICU staff would be asked to give tactful hints that the patient still has cardiac problems.

If I had unlimited resources, I would employ additional intensivists to do the aforementioned treatment, to titrate continuing care, to undertake supervision and training of residents, and to perform administrative duties. More critical care nurses would also be employed.

Patient B

Patient B's situation would not arise in our hospital. First, the emergency staff would not intubate the patient. Instead, staff from both the ICU and the internal medicine department would be consulted, and intubation would be discouraged. Second, admission to the ICU would be denied. The patient would be admitted to the medical ward, even if, by some error, he had been intubated. The internist would have primary responsibility for further care and for dealing with the patient's relatives. In all probability, the patient would be kept comfortable and noninvasive treatment such as antibiotic therapy would be provided. Third, bad news would likely not be given over the telephone to the patient's relatives; instead, they would be asked to come to the hospital. The family would then receive counseling, sympathy, and other psychosocial support.

In the great majority of cases, agreement with the medical assessment and plan is easily achieved. If conflict arises, which is rare, it is dealt with through the available channels of complaint. The internist would generally not reconsult the ICU staff and would handle the situation on the medical ward. If the patient did indeed turn around, the ICU staff might be reconsulted. In such a situation, it is likely that we would recommend continuation of current therapy, but ICU admission would probably still be denied. The ICU staff would instead review the patient's case serially on the ward and offer opinions on care as required.

If I had unlimited resources, my treatment would be the same.

Patient C

Patient C's situation would not arise in our hospital. A checklist of futile options, which would give false hope, would not be read to him. To do this to patients in a moribund condition in our social context would be deemed cruel. Staff from both the ICU and the surgery department would be consulted, and noninvasive treatment would be the consensus decision. Admission to ICU would be denied. The patient would thus be admitted to the surgical ward. The surgeon would have primary responsibility for further care. The patient would receive counseling, sympathy, and other psychosocial support. The surgeon would generally not reconsult the ICU staff and would handle the situation on the surgical ward, with consultations to other specialties for medical opinion as required. If invasive procedures were planned to control the bleeding, it is likely that the anesthesiologist would decline to provide anesthesia. The ICU would decline to provide postoperative support and would recommend postoperative return to the surgical ward, for comfort care if necessary.

If I had unlimited resources, my treatment would be the same.

Israel

Aviel Roy-Shapira, MD

Patient A

I think that Patient A has a grave prognosis, but his case is not hopeless. He sustained a witnessed arrest and presumably had effective cardiopulmonary resuscitation immediately. Therefore, he may not have anoxic brain damage. His pulmonary, renal, and hepatic functions are all reversible, individually, and his management until his admission was suboptimal. I believe that this patient ought to get the best that we have to offer. So for Patient A, it is easier to answer the second question first.

If I had free rein, here is what I would do: At the time of admission, the patient is in shock and has respiratory failure and renal failure. There is some question of hepatic dysfunction, and his neurological status is hard to gauge. We would need to address each problem, but by far the most important initially is the hemodynamic situation. It is quite possible that the renal and hepatic dysfunction would reverse if we were able to restore tissue perfusion.

The first order of business would be to get a better hemodynamic diagnosis. In our situation in Israel, the process of getting an echo-cardiogram is somewhat long; it takes at least 3 or 4 hours. A pulmonary artery catheter would be available immediately. Consequently, I would insert a pulmonary artery catheter, but I would obtain an echocardiogram as soon as possible. Although we are aware of the controversies around using these catheters, and I agree that they should not be used indiscriminately, in this case physical examination is inadequate. The hemodynamic profile would essentially determine management. If the filling pressures were high, we would start with an inotrope. My preference would be norepinephrine; dobutamine would also be a good choice. If there was no response, an aortic balloon might be indicated. I think, however, that the patient is hypovolemic. There are several indicators, such as his increased hemoglobin concentration. Judicious fluid challenges (crystalloids only) might be all that he needs. The key here would be to give small volumes, say 200 mL of lactated Ringer's solution every 15–20 minutes, and measure frequently.

This is problematic in Israel, because only doctors can do the measurements. This means that until the patient's perfusion was restored, I would need to sit on this patient. The issue of ventilation would need to be addressed. My immediate goal would be to reduce his FIO_2 to nontoxic levels. If the chest radiograph was from the referring hospital, I would request another, to make sure that there was no pneumothorax or large effusion. If there was none, I would begin pressure control ventilation and increase positive end-expiratory pressure (PEEP). With hemodynamic data available, I could increase PEEP to the inflection point without further compromising the patient's cardiac output. If we were successful at improving his hemodynamics, and renal function was not restored, or if he went into fluid overload, we would start continuous venovenous hemofiltration as renal replacement therapy.

I would not, at this time, give any antibiotics. I would do a mini–bronchoaveolar lavage as soon as the hemodynamics improved and would give antibiotics only when the results were positive. I believe that when one gives any drug, one carries the burden of proof that it does any good, and I found no evidence that giving any antibiotics in this situation changes the outcome. In a recent study in which brushes and mini–bronchoaveolar lavage were used, only a third of the patients with suspected aspiration or ventilator-associated pneumonia had a bacterial infection. Patients with bacterial pneumonia may benefit a little from earlier antibiotic treatment, but I believe that giving broad-spectrum antibiotics empirically actually makes us lose the Red Queen Race with the bacteria. Just like the Red Queen in Alice's looking glass world, in our war with the bugs we must run as fast as we can just to stay in the same place. When we give broad-spectrum antibiotics to patients who do not need it, we are going backward, because the practice gives free rein to *Candida* and other resistant organisms.

My answer to the first question is shorter. In general, we would manage the case as just outlined. However, I might not be able to get the hemodynamic measurements as often as I would like. We have a 12-bed unit, with a nurse-to-patient ratio of 1:2 (occasionally, particularly at night, 2:5). There are two residents in the house at night, but one of them answers trauma calls, and only one might be available. There is no 24-hour in-house attending, and it might not be possible to have a physician at the patient's bedside all the time. As I indicated earlier, only physicians take the hemodynamic profile. If the other patients in the ICU did not require constant physician attention, the patient would be managed according to plan. If another patient, perhaps with a better prognosis, needed similar attention, corners would be cut and the patient would probably die.

Patient B

Patient B is clearly dying. The proviso that he has no health care insurance is irrelevant in Israel; there is a national health insurance system and everyone is covered. As before, I think it is easier to answer question 2 first. If I had unlimited authority, I would discontinue mechanical ventilation and place the patient on morphine drip, with the aim of avoiding respiratory distress. I would let nature run its course.

There are three legitimate reasons to discontinue medical care. First, one can stop medical care because the patient does not want it. I do not think there is much dispute about that any longer. Second, one can stop medical care because resources are limited and it is necessary to decide whom to treat. The issue is that of allocation of resources. In general, I believe this is not a medical question but a political or social question. The community has to decide how it wants to distribute its resources. There should be open public discussion, and the conclusions should be in the public domain. It should not be part of the physician's decision-making process. I believe that the most ethical solution is to adopt a first-come-first-served policy; otherwise, one quickly starts judging who shall die and who shall live.

The third reason to discontinue medical care is that medical care is not indicated. Medical care may not be indicated for a variety of reasons. I do not like to use the term *futility,* because it is too vague. In Patient B's case, I believe that treatment would only prolong death and thus would do more harm than good. When medical care is not indicated, neither the wishes of the patient nor those of his relatives are relevant. This is a technical issue, and it is the decision of the physician alone. I therefore would not consult with the family but instead would explain what we planned to do. I think it is wrong and cruel to ask family members. It creates an unsolvable dilemma for them. Nobody wants to take responsibility for the death of a loved one. Nobody should. This stance is not paternalistic. It is not paternalistic to refuse to prescribe antibiotics for the common cold, regardless of the patient's wishes, and it is not paternalistic to refuse to operate when the risk of the operation outweighs the possible benefits. Similarly, it is not paternalistic to stop treatment when it can no longer accomplish its goals.

In actual practice, however, I would not discontinue ventilation. Instead, I would leave everything as is and not change any parameters. The result would be the same, except that death would occur about 24 hours later. The reasons behind my decision are local politics, peer pressure, and hospital policy. According to the Halakha, or Jewish law, it is forbidden to stop treatment. Even rabbis, however, understand that futile care is detrimental. There are several relevant examples in the Talmud. One such example involves a patient dying in his house. A woodcutter is chopping wood in the yard outside, and the loud noise prevents the soul from departing. The sages of the Talmud ruled that one should ask the woodcutter to stop the racket, so that the soul can depart in peace. One may conclude from this example that the Halakha recognizes that one ought to stop measures that only delay an inevitable death.

Recently, three of the most respected authorities in the Orthodox Jewish community issued a ruling that allows physicians not to stop medical care but to keep things as they are. This means that no laboratory studies are done, vital functions are not checked, no adjustments are made to the ventilator settings, inotrope doses are not increased or decreased, and no new drugs are added. Only a standard maintenance schedule of fluids and painkillers, as necessary, can be followed. The effect of this policy was studied in a hospital in Jerusalem, where the majority of patients belong to the ultra-Orthodox community. The researchers found that all patients invariably died within 48 hours. Because this approach is accepted by the Orthodox community, it is also accepted by hospital administrations. I really have little say in the matter, if I want to keep my job. In Patient B's case, the extra time in the unit puts little burden on the nurses and other medical staff, so it is not worth a big argument. Occasionally we run into trouble, when the bed is required for another patient. In that case, I would have to involve the hospital medical director, who might authorize transfer of the patient, ventilated, to a regular hospital floor.

Patient C

When treatment is futile, the patient's wishes are irrelevant. I am not obligated to deliver the futile care; it is actually my duty to refrain. Suppose a patient with metastatic pancreatic cancer demanded a Whipple operation because his rabbi promised him a miracle, provided we the surgeons helped God a little by removing the primary. I would not do the operation for all the money in world (to be honest, *all* the money in the world might cloud my judgment some, but it would have to be a very large sum indeed before I succumbed to the temptation). I believe I have a moral duty to deny futile care, regardless of the patient's demands. My problem is that I am not sure treatment in Patient C's case would be futile. To explain why, let me review his current situation.

He has massive upper gastrointestinal bleeding but maintains adequate cerebral perfusion; he is completely lucid. Thus he is still able to compensate for the hypovolemia. So in spite of the oozing blood, he is not in deep shock. Moreover, I cannot assume that he is bleeding from varices. At least half of these patients bleed from other sources, some of which are easily controlled endoscopically, such as a duodenal ulcer. Even if it is from varices, one can often stop the bleeding with sclerotherapy or rubber band ligation, or, as a last resort, a transjugular intrahepatic portosystemic shunt.

The patient also has obvious liver cirrhosis, with a degree of acute liver failure, but no ascites and no encephalopathy. The latter is particularly significant. Massive gastrointestinal bleeding usually worsens any existing encephalopathy and may be the trigger for its first appearance. So the lack thereof in this patient indicates that the liver is not completely burned out. It is possible, and even likely, that his jaundice and loss of synthetic function are due to some acute condition, most probably ethanol-induced hepatitis. If this is the case, there is a substantial chance that it is reversible.

This man also has acquired immunodeficiency syndrome (AIDS), the actual state of which is unknown, but there is no evidence of sepsis at this time. It is said that he does not comply with his medications, but this is uncertain.

All this is present in a patient who is engaged in self-destructive activities and is recalcitrant. There is a little chance that he will rehabilitate himself. However, this seems to be his first real brush with death. It may have a sobering effect (pun intended), if he pulls through. In view of these considerations, I cannot rule that treatment would be futile. Under certain conditions, we could restore this patient to his previous state of health. The effect might be short-term. He could come next week with another similar episode (which might change my attitude), but then again, he could live happily for a few months, or maybe a year or two. I think that is a worthy goal. After all, physicians subject patients with incurable cancer to palliative operations and procedures and think nothing of it.

To judge that the life of this patient is not worth living is making a quality-of-life decision. I do not think that physicians should be allowed to make quality-of-life decisions. Having made these observations, I am ready to answer the two questions. In this case, the answer is the same for both. Broadly speaking, I would like to give this patient the benefit of the doubt. I am not sure that treatment would be futile, and I would need more time. I would admit the patient to the unit. Naturally, the usual delirium tremens precautions would be taken, and he would receive thiamine and mild sedation with midazolam. I would be quite happy with his blood pressure, but I would want to increase his hemoglobin concentration to about 7 or 8 g/dL. I would also transfuse fresh frozen plasma and other components to correct the coagulation profile. I would have a gastroscopy done as soon as possible to determine the source of bleeding. If the bleeding source was a duodenal ulcer, I would treat him aggressively for the remainder of his stay.

If the source was esophageal varices, I would attempt rubber band ligation or sclerotherapy. If the bleeding did not stop, we would have to reconsider, but I might insert a Sengstaken-Blakemore tube. Because of his AIDS and continued addiction, he is obviously not a candidate for transplantation, so I would not do a transjugular intrahepatic portosystemic shunt, and I also would not do a surgical shunt, because his operative mortality now is 100%. Consequently, if the bleeding continued, I would probably conclude that further care was futile and I would then provide comfort measures only.

To summarize, I think that with this patient, as described, one cannot initially rule that medical care is futile. It is possible that simple measures, such as those outlined here, would return him to his premorbid state. But the decision-making process is a dynamic one. If he continued to bleed, or if his condition deteriorated further, treatment would become futile and should then be stopped.

Canada

Ted S. Rogovein, MD

Patient A

Patient A has been admitted to our medical-surgical intensive care unit (ICU) from an institution unable to deal with his case. This man has multiple organ dysfunction that at this point is almost certainly reversible. Once transfer from the sending institution was completed, we would begin our stabilization by attempting to improve his organ dysfunction status. Although I will present the therapies in a linear fashion, most of these interventions would begin simultaneously.

This patient has developed acute respiratory distress syndrome (ARDS) secondary to aspiration of gastric contents. His oxygen saturation is 88% while he is receiving ventilation with an FIO_2 of 100% and a positive end-expiratory pressure (PEEP) of 5 cm H_2O. The mode of ventilation is not specified. This patient meets the criteria for ARDS, and we would elect to ventilate him according to the Acute Respiratory Distress Syndrome Clinical Network (ARDSNet) protocol and use volume ventilation with a tidal volume of 5–6 mL/kg of ideal body weight. Positive end-expiratory pressure would be increased, and we would try to decrease FIO_2. The patient would receive sedation and analgesia to aid with ventilation.

The patient is almost certainly volume contracted and would begin receiving crystalloid boluses immediately. It is unlikely that fluids alone would be adequate to increase this man's blood pressure and aid organ perfusion. We would likely start a norepinephrine infusion and attempt to increase his mean arterial pressure to 65–70 mm Hg while continuing crystalloid boluses or infusion.

The evidence for use of a pulmonary artery catheter in such cases is still pending. However, we would use a pulmonary artery catheter to aid us in our fluid and vasopressor management. This patient is having multifocal premature ventricular contractions and he has coagulopathy, so placement of the pulmonary artery catheter is not without major risk. However, I believe that following the trends of the data obtained using the pulmonary artery catheter would be helpful, and therefore one would be placed.

Given the patient's coagulopathy, we would also include fresh frozen plasma among the fluids used in resuscitation.

Continuous venovenous hemodiafiltration would be initiated after a nephrology consultation, if the nephrologist concurred. Cardiological opinion would also be obtained to aid with treatment of the patient's arrhythmias and to help assess left ventricular ejection fraction.

The choice of a first-generation cephalosporin to treat aspiration pneumonia is not one we would have made. Given the 3 days of sepsis in another institution, we would have chosen a wider spectrum of antimicrobials. We would begin empirically with an antipseudomonal agent as well as antibiotics against methicillin-resistant *Staphylococcus aureus* and anaerobes. Blood, urine, and sputum samples would be sent for culture.

If oxygenation or ventilation worsened while ARDSNet tidal volumes were used, we would consider therapy with high-frequency oscillation and/or nitric oxide (aware as we are of the need for evidence of efficacy for these interventions).

If the patient's hemodynamic status worsened, we would consider adding other inotropes or vasopressors as necessary, and if we thought doing so would be beneficial, we would insert an intra-aortic balloon pump.

The patient's neurological status is probably related to his overall septic state; however, if his level of consciousness did not improve, we would obtain a neurology consultation and obtain a computed tomography scan of his head.

The 25th-anniversary edition of *Maclean's* included the results of the magazine's annual poll of what values Canadians hold dear. According to the article, Canada's health care system, Medicare, remains "a matter of enormous pride for many Canadians, up there with the Maple Leaf flag as a symbol of what we are as a people."[1] The author and I share amazement that Medicare plays such an important role in Canadian self-identity, considering that the system has been around for only about 30 of Canada's 133 years. The federal legislation that codifies the five principles of the country's public health system, the Canada Health Act,[2] has been in existence only since 1985. These five principles are public administration, comprehensiveness, universality, portability, and accessibility. This system for ensuring that all Canadians have access to health care functions well for the most part. However, access to needed resources can at times be frustratingly slow. Waiting lists for certain procedures and technologies are longer than most patients and their health care workers would wish. With regard to Patient A, if I had unlimited access to resources and unlimited authority, I would have more rapid access to those resources.

Although Canadians are insured for 100% of their health care, some people never bother to obtain the documentation necessary for enrollment in the program. These individuals still receive full medical care; however, reimbursement for services rendered to such patients is often delayed and not always fully retroactive.

Visitors to Canada are not covered, nor are refugees (until their hearings begin, and then the federal government reimburses the provincial health care system).

If Patient A is a Canadian or is having his refugee status assessed, our taxes cover his care. However, whether Patient A is a Canadian or not, he should (and almost certainly would) receive the exact same level of care. Obviously, most Canadian physicians hope to be paid for their work, but this still would not change the care Patient A received. Although one would prefer that Canadians receive the health care that their taxes pay for (rather than nonresidents who do not pay taxes), the reality is that the acuity of the patient's condition and the potential reversibility of his underlying disease outweigh other factors.

Patient B

Patient B's premorbid status was quite poor. At age 88 years, he has a number of chronic diseases, including dementia, and he has required 24-hour nasal oxygen. This patient has now developed sepsis with shock. The patient was intubated and ventilated, with central access obtained and fluid resuscitation started, because relatives were called and said they wanted everything done. Patient B then developed multiple organ dysfunction with volume overload, pulmonary edema, and renal failure with hyperkalemia and metabolic acidosis.

Unfortunately, this is not an uncommon situation. People not skilled in critical care have little or no understanding of what "doing everything" entails, and I therefore believe that the phrase is a meaningless one. However, once resuscitation has been initiated because of the demand that everything be done, it is very difficult to suddenly stop therapy.

I would give the patient a 50-mL ampule of 50% dextrose intravenously and intravenous insulin and calcium to temporarily deal with the potential for cardiac arrhythmia related to the hyperkalemia. However, my most important intervention would be my discussions with family members. This superficial desire for everything to be done would have to be clarified. Although I would suggest to them that the outcome of any intervention was likely to be extremely poor, I would undertake a short trial of aggressive therapy to see if he indeed would improve as he had in the past. I would give the family an artificial timeline of 2–3 days for seeing if there was any improvement. This timeline would be a "floating window": I would tell the family members that if the patient showed continuing improvement, we would continue our aggressive therapy for another 2–3 days, and we would continually reassess.

This patient will require dialysis if he is going to survive in the short term. A nephrology consultation would be obtained and acute dialysis started. Acute dialysis in this type of situation is not difficult to initiate. However, there is a shortage of chronic dialysis spaces in Toronto and the surrounding cities. Given his multitude of chronic diseases, his advanced age, and his dementia, it is unlikely that this patient would be accepted for chronic dialysis. Both the nephrologist and I would clearly outline for the family the plan for acute intervention with no intention of chronic dialysis.

Vasopressor therapy would be started, and the patient would be made comfortable with analgesia and sedation. Blood, urine, and sputum cultures would be obtained, and treatment with broad-spectrum antibiotics would be started, with kidney-toxic choices being avoided. I would not insert a pulmonary artery catheter but would transduce the central line and follow his central venous pressure trend. I suspect that his infiltrates and oxygen status would improve with ultrafiltration, but I would increase PEEP while waiting for this improvement. If his infiltrates did not improve with ultra-filtration, he would be ventilated using ARDSNet-protocol volume-based ventilation.

I would head the multidisciplinary team that would have daily meetings with the family, meetings in which the present situation and the prognosis would be emphasized. If the patient responded to our inter-ventions, we would continue our therapy for another 2–3 days. However, if he showed no improvement over those 2–3 days, or if he deteriorated despite our aggressive measures, we would recommend to the family a change in focus from aggressive measures to comfort measures.

In our experience, the vast majority of families are reasonable about this change in focus, especially if the physician has made an earnest attempt to reverse the acute disease process and has kept the family involved and aware of the situation.

There are, of course, families who continue to insist on aggressive measures even in the most hopeless of situations, in which deterioration continues despite therapies. Although they constitute a minority, it is these families that critical care personnel tend to remember and focus on. This is very understandable, because the situation tends to be a most frustrating experience for all concerned. We usually require regular protracted family meetings and involve the chaplain, request an ethics consultation, and obtain a second (and third) critical care physician opinion. We also suggest that the family ask a trusted physician to discuss the case with us. Again, portions of these families do eventually come to terms with the situation and allow the dying process to conclude without further prolongation.

Despite all this information, there will be families who will not see the circumstances as the medical team does and will not agree to a change in focus of care. If Patient B's family belonged to this small minority of "vitalists," we would continue our attempts to keep the lines of communication open and would make sure the family understood that the patient was likely to die despite our present interventions. In such cases, we do end up prolonging the dying process, even though the family cannot recognize this. I do not add any new therapies in these situations unless they are for the comfort of the patient. Cardiopulmonary resuscitation is not performed when it will not work (such as in Patient B's case), and this is explained to the family. The option of transfer of the patient to another institution is given to these families but is rarely accepted.

I do not believe that there would be much change in the way I would treat Patient B if his family was like the majority of families I routinely encounter in my ICU. If I had unlimited resources and unlimited authority, the only major change in care for this patient would be strict enforcement of my set timeline if the patient's family belonged to that small subset of families who are vitalists.

Although I appreciate that it can take time for some people to come to terms with the impending death of a loved one, I also believe that once death is almost certain, it is inappropriate to prolong the dying process. If Patient B's situation was not improving or was deteriorating beyond my original set time limit, I would begin comfort measures and withdraw aggressive care. I further believe that cardiac arrest secondary to multiple organ failure in a patient with such a poor premorbid health status is a terminal event. If I had unlimited authority, unreasonable and ineffective interventions such as cardiopulmonary resuscitation would not be offered to this patient. As well, once it became clear that the patient was not going to survive, the focus of care would be palliation, with a plan to transfer him to a palliative care unit.

Patient C

Patient C is dying and has no hope of recovery. One could choose any prognostic scoring system one wished; however, the bedside assessment of this patient is clear: he is going to die, and no therapy is going to change that outcome. Patient C should not have been read options to pick from; patient care possibilities should not be presented like some restaurant menu. He should have been told that our plan was to make sure that he was comfortable, and that he would receive aggressive comfort care on a ward, not in the ICU. This patient does not fit criteria for admission to our ICU; he is preterminal with irreversible disease. I would have involved our palliative care team and human immunodeficiency virus (HIV) specialists in this patient's care. His lack of relatives, alcohol abuse, HIV status, lack of insurance, and history of noncompliance are not issues here. He has every right to ask for another opinion, another physician to be in charge of his care, or transferral to another institution. He does not have the right to ICU admission simply because he wishes everything done, just as he would not be offered a liver or lung transplantation if he wished one and the organ was available. Whether I had unlimited resources and unlimited authority or not would have no effect on the underlying inappropriateness of admitting this irreversibly ill patient to anywhere other than a palliative care setting. If "doing everything" has any meaning at all, that meaning probably is "do not abandon this patient."

References

[1]Marshall R: Paying the price. Maclean's. December 25, 2000.
[2]RS 1985, c C-6. Also available at: http://laws.justice.gc.ca/en/C-6/text.html. Accessed September 24, 2001.

Urban United States

Don Chalfin, MD

Patient A

On transfer of Patient A to the intensive care unit (ICU), or perhaps on initial evaluation by the critical care physician, the first task would be to stabilize the patient and focus on his many concurrent multisystem life-threatening processes. In view of his cardiac events and low perfusional state, the first priority concerns his cardiogenic shock, because his hemo-dynamic insufficiency requires immediate stabilization with aggressive fluid infusions along with vasopressors and other related therapies. An indwelling arterial catheter should be inserted, and strong consideration would also be given to the expeditious placement of a pulmonary artery catheter for diagnostic purposes and assessment of therapeutic efficacy, in view of his myocardial damage and tenuous cardiac status, low urine output, increased heart rate, and increased blood urea nitrogen and creatinine levels.

Once his cardiac status was stabilized, immediate attention could then be focused on his tenuous respiratory status—as evidenced by an oxygen saturation of 88% despite 100% FIO_2 and 5 cm H_2O of positive end-expiratory pressure. His physiological parameters and ventilatory status would be carefully assessed. It is likely that his ventilator settings would have to be adjusted to optimize his pulmonary status and minimize potential adverse sequelae in the face of aspiration and acute respiratory distress syndrome (ARDS). If oxygenation did not improve, consideration might also be given to alternative modes of ventilatory support, including pressure control and inverse ratio ventilation.

Throughout this process of assessment and stabilization of the patient's hemodynamic and pulmonary processes, attention would also be given to his other afflicted systems and concurrent and interrelated problems, including his neurological status, renal failure, coagulopathy, leukocytosis, and likely septic sequelae.

This patient would be best served by a critical care specialist who would direct the care and supervise all clinical actions. However, in urban America, provision of critical care services is quite variable and often reflects institutional, specialty, and even personal bias. In the best-case scenario, an intensivist would be at the scene as soon as the problems became evident, would be continuously present at the bedside until the patient stabilized, and would be constantly available. He or she would administer the fluids and vasopressors, insert (or supervise the insertion of) the arterial line and the pulmonary artery catheter, assess and interpret the pulmonary parameters and adjust the ventilator and the mode of mechanical ventilation, and essentially assume responsibility for all clinical decisions and become the point person for all involved clinicians and even for the patient and his family during the ICU course.

However, this model for critical care delivery is not the norm in urban America. Many scenarios for the delivery of critical care services exist, yet the common feature of most is the presence of multiple consultants called on behalf of the primary care physician or the attending of record, each one addressing his or her area of expertise. In Patient A's case, the cardiologist might be the person who inserts the pulmonary artery catheter and could even serve as the one who decides among the various antiarrhythmics, inotropes, and vasopressors. A pulmonary specialist would be called to manage the ventilator and to consult about the ARDS and aspiration. An infectious disease physician might also be involved, especially if the patient continued to exhibit leukocytosis and manifest signs of sepsis. In addition, a nephrologist would be asked to provide input regarding the azotemia and the decreased urinary output. It is also likely that a hematology consultation would be requested, given the patient's coagulopathy, and a gastro-enterologist and/or liver specialist might be solicited for advice as well, in view of the transaminitis. It is important to recognize that although consul-tants usually attempt to contact the physician of record and keep him or her informed of their impressions and actions, they often work independently of one another in an episodic fashion.

With respect to involvement by a critical care practitioner, the pulmonary physician will often have expertise and perhaps even board certification in critical care; however, in all too many cases, he or she focuses only on the respiratory system and defers other problems to the cadre of other consultants. In almost all other cases, a critical care physician—a physician separate from the pulmonary specialist—may be involved; however, the extent of this involvement will vary.

In the best-case scenario, with expenditure of unlimited resources on the basis of the best available evidence that the outcome will justify the expense, and with freedom from political constraints and reimbursement concerns, a critical care physician would likely be able to assume primary responsibility as described. However, in the real-world setting of urban America, a critical care physician will often be called for consultation only at the request of the primary physician; in this way, the critical care physician is akin to other consulting physicians. Furthermore, it is entirely likely that the critical care physician, as a consultant, will be asked to offer his or her services and expertise not when the critical conditions begin but when they become apparent to the attending physician. The intensivist may also serve a role with regard to ICU triage and bed clearance and access issues and may see the patient only during teaching rounds with the housestaff assigned to the ICU. As a consultant, the intensivist may need to collaborate with the other physicians involved in the patient's care. These variable models of critical care notwithstanding, more and more hospitals, physicians, and health care professionals are recognizing the services that a qualified critical care physician can provide. It is therefore anticipated that patients like Patient A will be increasingly cared for by qualified critical care practitioners at the onset of and throughout their critical illnesses.

Patient B

In the best-case scenario in urban America, with resources plentiful, clinical restraints minimal, and reimbursement and political concerns nonexistent, a critical care physician would be immediately on the scene to care for Patient B. He or she would not only direct the clinical issues but also supervise and institute comfort measures as well as oversee all issues related to end-of-life and ethical concerns. In all issues related to the patient's critical illness and multisystem dysfunction, the critical care physician would serve as the captain of the team, soliciting the involvement and expertise of all team members and even expanding the team roster when other expertise was warranted. The intensivist would manage the patient's cardiogenic insufficiency and ventilatory dysfunction and would, as with the first case, perform all procedures; interpret all physiological data; order most (perhaps all) diagnostic tests; administer all fluids, vasopressors, and vasoactive agents; and coordinate all aspects of the patient's care. Furthermore, it is entirely likely that the intensivist would be involved at the outset, when the patient first arrived at the emergency department, and not merely come on the scene when the patient presented to the ICU.

In this setting, the intensivist would also concurrently serve as the primary conduit and contact point for the patient's family. Patient B has no living will, and the family has expressed a desire to have everything done, despite the patient's moribund condition. Clearly, this represents a difficult situation, but it is one that is common to practicing intensivists. Yet in this scenario, when constraints are few and resources are many, the intensivist has the opportunity to establish a relationship with the family and work toward a humane and reasoned resolution that factors in the family's concerns and the patient's grave prognosis. This idealized scenario portrays a paradox, in which the intensivist is able to provide the appropriate level of clinical care and patient supervision but must balance this against ethical and futility issues. However, in this scenario, the chances are significantly higher that the patient will receive the maximal level of care as expertly and expeditiously as possible, but only while a potential benefit still exists.

In the more realistic setting that characterizes medical care in urban America, it is likely that the care would be fragmented among many physicians and many consultants. An intensivist might be involved, however, as with the first patient; the involvement would vary from hospital to hospital and even from unit to unit. Many clinical decisions would have to be deferred to the primary attending and the other consultants, especially when they impinged on another physician's expertise and organ-specific "domain." However, the major issues in this case that are likely to be affected revolve around the ethical, compassionate care, and end-of-life questions. Because the attending physician of record assumes ultimate responsibility, final decisions will fall within his or her domain or at least will require his or her agreement and final approval. Yet all too often, the attending physician is removed from the pressing clinical issues relating to critically ill patients. The attending physician is usually present at the patient's bedside for only brief periods, may be unable to recognize the complex interrelationships inherent in the treatment of critically ill patients, and may even lack familiarity with the patient and his or her family (in Patient B's case, because of the presence of long-standing chronic illnesses and residence in a nursing home). Thus it may be difficult to communicate the gravity of the patient's current clinical condition to the family and develop an ethical plan that factors in the futility and comfort care issues.

In consultation-driven medicine, patients are likely to receive expensive and aggressive interventions even when potential benefit is no longer evident. The absence of a captain in the critical care setting further exacerbates this clinical fragmentation. In addition, such an absence may serve as a shield for all involved physicians, preventing or at least impeding them from addressing the overriding ethical concerns and determining appropriate clinical limits. The presence of a critical care practitioner and an active critical care service would clearly serve to minimize and even eliminate these barriers, but only if the intensivist was empowered to act independently, proactively, and decisively.

Patient C

Urban American hospitals continually deal with large numbers of patients with problems related to acquired immunodeficiency syndrome (AIDS) and human immunodeficiency virus infection and/or problems and diseases related to drug and alcohol abuse. Many such patients highlight the disparities in American medicine, because they often lack health insurance and access to standard primary care services and related preventive necessities. Although many of these patients receive care from free clinics, charitable organizations, municipal and Veterans Affairs hospitals, and tertiary care medical institutions, clearly the haves and have-nots often receive different care. Poor or absent indemnity coverage has an impact on patient health and access to medical care. In addition, hospitals that treat a large number of uninsured patients often face severe financial pressure and budgetary crises, because of their legal and moral obligations to provide care for these patients.

In this particular case, if resources were plentiful and constraints— both political and financial—were minimal, Patient C would receive expeditious care commensurate with his condition. In all probability, a critical care physician would be immediately involved in his care and would assume primary clinical responsibility for the pressing clinical decisions related to his critical illness. If other consultants were required, they would be quickly called, regardless of the patient's insurance and payer status; medical necessity and medical necessity alone would determine the level of care and the services rendered. Accordingly, the patient would undergo all tests whenever needed and would also have surgery or other interventional procedures should his condition warrant. In this world of limitless resources and equal access, no financial barriers or "needs test" would exist. Furthermore, it is entirely likely that the this patient would present quite differently and perhaps less dramatically (if at all), because he would have stood a greater chance of receiving comprehensive primary care and preventive services, including alcohol and drug treatment and even comprehensive AIDS management, approaches that could increase his understanding of his health and disease and thereby improve his compliance.

In the realistic, resource-constrained world of urban America, however, a different scenario and different course of events would unfold. In many and perhaps most situations, the patient would likely be admitted by a "service" attending or a rotating attending physician assigned to admit such patients under his or her clinical service. In teaching hospitals, the housestaff often manages these "service" patients, with little or no supervision by the attending of record. Similarly, hospitals that care for large numbers of uninsured and indigent patients often lack valuable resources, in part because of the high level of unreimbursed and under-reimbursed care, but also because of the inability to attract the physicians and the clinical expertise necessary for state-of-the-art programs. With respect to patients like Patient C, another dichotomy might arise when the expertise of other specialists is required, because some physicians might be reluctant to provide consultations, given the lack of health insurance and the slim chance for meaningful remuneration.

Finally, although these social and financial barriers exert a profound impact on all aspects of Patient C's hospitalization, both in and out of the ICU, the indirect impact may be even greater, given the increased likelihood of reduced preventive care and proactive interventions that could have attenuated his disease processes in the first place, thereby attenuating his need for ICU care and hospitalization at this juncture.

Summaries of
Medical Comments

Patient A

Is Treatment Worthwhile?

Bruce Gipe, MD

Patient A is in good company in the United States. About 1.5 million patients experience acute myocardial infarction annually, and about $60 billion is spent on care for this disease each year.[1] In 1995, about 1.6 million cardiac catheterizations were performed in the United States; this number is expected to increase to 3 million by 2010.[2] In 1997, approximately 170,000 angioplasty procedures were performed in the Medicare population alone.[3] About 44 million Americans are, like Patient A, uninsured.

A good clinical outcome for Patient A should make him a poster child for the efficacy of critical care medicine. His cardiac arrest occurred during an invasive procedure in the cardiac catheterization suite, and his subsequent illness (respiratory failure due to development of acute respiratory distress syndrome) is an event that results in about 100,000 intensive care unit (ICU) admissions per year in the United States,[4] providing critical care physicians and nurses with ample opportunity to demonstrate their best skills.

If critical care did not exist, Patient A would quickly die after his initial resuscitation from a second cardiac arrest that would be caused by hypoxemia. Society has decided to support the infrastructure of critical care, giving Patient A the opportunity to survive his illness and return to productivity.

Patient A not only is desperately ill but also might respond to salvage treatment, despite the fact that two organ systems (the respiratory and renal systems) have failed and a third organ system (the central nervous system) is in question. On top of that, he has just experienced an acute coronary event. If he survives and returns to work, he will do so only because he has received excellent care from skilled clinicians who understand how to manage his pulmonary, renal, and cardiac status while supporting the function of his brain.

A Direct-Cost Estimate

A finite number of dollars will be spent to pull Patient A through. Presented in Table 1 is an estimate of the costs that would be incurred over the first 4 days of intensive care at the referring facility. Patient A's first 4 days of care resulted in approximately $27,000 in direct costs.

Table 1. Approximate direct cost of care for Patient A at referring facility, days 1–4

	Facility cost	Physician cost*
Day 1		
Emergency department		
Room	$250	
Electrocardiogram		$12
Laboratory	$200	
X-ray	$100	$50
Pharmacy	$300	
Supplies	$100	
Emergency physician		$168
Cardiologist		$220
Subtotal	*$950*	*$450*
Angiography suite		
Room	$1,689*	
Supplies	$500	
Pharmacy	$250	
Cardiologist		$1,469
Anesthesiologist		$500
Subtotal	*$2,439*	*$1,969*
Cardiac care unit		
Room	$1,295	
Pharmacy	$350	
Laboratory	$265	
X-ray	$140	
Supplies	$325	
Respiratory care	$125	
Subtotal	*$2,500*	
Days 2–4		
Room ($2500/d)	$7,500	
Cardiologist		$660
Pulmonologist		$544
Infectious disease specialist		$370
Helicopter	$10,000	
Subtotal	*$17,500*	*$1,574*
Total	**$23,389**	**$3,993**

*2001 Medicare Fee Schedule for Area 18.

Having arrived at a tertiary facility that is capable of delivering some combination of services described previously by the physicians from 11 countries, Patient A starts on a tedious but inexorably successful road to recovery. Presented in Table 2 is a direct cost estimate for the next 30 days of acute care, followed by 30 days of subacute care, followed by 15 days of care in a skilled nursing facility.

Table 2. Estimated costs of ongoing care for Patient A

	Cost
Intensive care unit ($2,500/d)	$37,500
Intermediate care ($1,000/d)	$5,000
Medical-surgical care ($500/d)	$5,000
Care and consultations, by physician	
Intensivist	$2,370
Nephrologist	$660
Neurologist	$778
Infectious disease specialist	$840
Hospitalist	$930
Procedures	
Tracheostomy	$289
Chest tube	$258
Dialysis ($152/d)	$760
Pulmonary artery catheter	$177
Arterial catheter	$65
Subacute unit	
Room ($400/d)	$12,000
Skilled nursing unit	
Room ($200/d)	$3,000
Total	**$69,627**

Patient A, after spending 75 days in health care facilities and incurring total estimated direct costs of $97,009, has returned home. He now requires 30 days of outpatient physical therapy. A speech therapist also is required, because of his moderate vocal cord injury. After this period, his tracheostomy stoma is healed, his blood pressure is well controlled, he is experiencing no chest pain, he is walking 2 miles a day, and he feels he can return to work as the assistant sales manager at a local automobile tire dealership.

Society's Contribution to Patient A's Costs

Patient A has no health insurance. In California, he would not qualify for the state's Medicaid program (Medi-Cal), because he is not elderly (at least 65 years old), blind, or disabled (for a period of at least 1 year). In the mid 1980s, when California was experiencing a recession, the state legislature eliminated the Medically Indigent Adult Program. This program had become extremely costly ($800 million per year in 1983, $2 billion per year if it were to be reimplemented in 2001), and huge savings were achieved by dropping about 300,000 people from its rolls (P. Abbott, oral communication, April 2001). When this happened, the financial responsibility for the care of indigent patients such as Patient A was shifted to the counties and the providers.

In 2000, the California Medical Association estimated that physicians alone absorbed $400 million in unpaid claims for care provided to California's indigent residents (approximately $5300 per licensed California physician). Currently, 34 counties in California administer a fund for the care of their indigent residents who do not qualify for Medi-Cal. Some of these funds derive from Proposition 99 tobacco tax revenues, and payments from these funds are meted out in proportion to the ratio of the total dollars in the fund at the end of the year to the total claims received (e.g., if the fund has $1 million and the claims of an individual county make up 10% of the total claims made during the year, the county would receive $100,000 from the fund). In 17 of California's 58 counties, actual county hospitals exist and provide acute care services, allowing the noncounty, private hospitals to refer patients to them and therefore avoid the expenses associated with the care of the indigent.

In some states, Patient A would qualify for Medicaid. The Medicaid program was created along with the Medicare program in 1965 as part of President Johnson's Great Society. It is now the largest health insurance program in the United States, covering services for about 41 million people.[5] In 1997, approximately $160 billion was expended on the Medicaid program in the United States. The federal share of this amount was $95 billion, and the individual states contributed $65 billion. The 2001 Medi-Cal budget is about $25 billion. Approximately 51% of this amount will be paid by the federal government, and the rest will come from the state's general fund. The Medi-Cal program pays physicians about 30% of the Medicare fees for inpatient care. The program pays hospitals about 40% of their usual and customary charges.

Unfortunately for Patient A, Medicaid eligibility is not directly linked to a certain level of income. In 1997, only 44% of nonelderly persons with an income of less than $13,330 (the federal poverty level for a family of three) were covered by Medicaid. The working poor make up the largest portion of the uninsured in the United States, a group that now represents about 16% of the entire population. If Patient A returns to work, retires at age 65, and dies from an acute myocardial infarction at age 70, society will have spent an additional $51,000 (given 1997 per capita expenditures for health care equal to $3925)[6] or more on health care for Patient A.

Patient A's Contribution to His Health Care Costs

If Patient A qualifies for Medicaid, and if Medicaid pays the hospitals 40% of their costs, society will actually spend about $37,690 for his hospital costs. If Medicaid pays the physicians 30% of their fees, society will actually spend approximately $3300 on his physician component of care. This means that the hospital will have to absorb about $51,500 in direct costs and the physicians will absorb about $8000.

It is possible to estimate the amount of money that Patient A has contributed to his health care via taxation. For example, it is known that individuals born in 1945 will over their working lifetimes have paid taxes to support Medicare that range from $38,000 to $120,000 (in 1990 dollars and depending on their levels of income).[7] A couple retiring in 1998, with one wage earner having paid taxes for 32 years, would have paid $16,790 into the Medicare program.[8] Medicare Part A is supported through a 2.9% income tax (one-half paid by the employee and one-half paid by the employer); Medicare Part B funds come mostly from general tax revenues that are appropriated by Congress, along with a monthly premium ($43.80 in 1998) that is paid by beneficiaries. If Patient A currently earns $18,500 per year, has been paying income taxes since he began working at age 17, and has had an average income of $15,000, he has paid about $9000 (1.45% × $15,000/year × 40 years) into the Medicare Part A program.

However, Patient A does not qualify for the Medicare program, because he is less than 65 years old, is not disabled, and does not have end-stage renal disease. He has contributed indirectly to his health care costs via tax payments, at the federal and state levels, that were used to fund his state's Medicaid program and/or local funding programs for the indigent. Using tax tables published by the Internal Revenue Service, one can estimate the amount of federal income tax paid by Patient A over his lifetime, by adjusting the per capita tax figures that are provided. For example, the year 2000 tax schedules show that Patient A would owe about $2200 in federal income tax. The per capita tax payment in 1998 averaged $6521.[9] Using the ratio of $2200 to $6521 and calculating back to 1961 when Patient A first began to pay taxes, one finds that the total amount paid would be about $38,000. Thus, even if all of Patient A's tax payments were stored in a lockbox to pay for his health care, society would need to come up with additional funds to fully compensate his providers for the current episode of care.

Is It Worthwhile to Treat Patient A?

In the previous section, I demonstrated that society has paid out far more than Patient A has paid in for his health care. This imbalance highlights the conflict between limited resources and unlimited demand for health care. In June 2000, the United States Supreme Court, in *Pegram v. Herdich,*[10] faced this same issue and acknowledged that "the profit incentive to ration care" exists and is legal. In so doing, the Court recognized the fact that physicians do play a dual role, functioning both as clinicians and as "benefits administrators."[11]

In the Herdich case, a patient in Illinois sued her health plan for offering financial rewards to physicians to limit care (she alleged that for financial reasons, an abdominal ultrasound was not ordered and that this delayed the diagnosis of acute appendicitis, resulting in peritonitis). According to one author, the Court's ruling in this case "summoned Americans to confront the conflict between health care cost consciousness and insistence, when ill, on all that medicine might offer."[11]

Patient A was not covered by a managed care plan with incentives for its physicians to limit care in light of his high mortality risk (given essentially two failed organ systems). One must consider whether there are other incentives to limit care that would allow society to avoid "cost overruns" that result from providing services to Patient A and the rest of the uninsured population. If, for example, in the year that Patient A is being treated, the tertiary hospital experiences unanticipated decreases in revenue or increases in expenses, causing it to close entirely or to shut down certain services to avoid closure or bankruptcy, one could argue that a program to limit access to critical care on the basis of mortality prediction would be justifiable.

From 1995 to 1999, the number of American hospitals decreased by 6.4% because of closures. In 1999, there were 5890 hospitals in the United States, and in that year there were 190 hospital closures.[12] The Medicare Payment Advisory Committee recently reported that hospitals with negative total margins reached their highest percentage in a decade, up to 34% in 1998.[12] One consulting firm estimated that by 2004, a total of 60% of all hospitals in the United States will be losing money.[13] Likewise, if the clinicians involved in providing care for Patient A found at the end of the year that their expenses exceeded revenue, then rationing care to focus on patients who are more likely to survive could make sense, to avoid an ensuing loss of providers. The California Medical Association and Pricewaterhouse-Coopers reported in 1999 that two of three medical groups in California were losing money, that 8 of 10 groups could not meet basic financial benchmarks, and that 1 in 10 groups was expected to fail.[14]

Proper resource allocation in the ICU demands a consideration of profound clinical and ethical issues. In a recent report on patient's perspectives concerning good-quality end-of-life care, the need to avoid "inappropriate prolongation of dying" was identified as one of five principal areas of concern in a sample of dialysis patients, people with human immuno-deficiency virus infection, and residents of a long-term-care facility.[15] Currently, there is no uniform standard that can be used to determine whether use of an ICU bed is appropriate for a given condition. Community standards for the extremes of illness and injury are generally effective with regard to provision of care to patients with acute respiratory failure, acute myocardial infarction, and shock. The development of "chest pain centers" has helped to unload the patient who is stable, and awaiting the results of cardiac enzyme tests, from the ICU to the emergency department or step-down unit.

At the other end of the intensive care spectrum—patients with stays longer than 14 days—costs and outcomes have also been scrutinized. Of 690 patients admitted to a medical-surgical ICU at a tertiary hospital in Canada, 9% had ICU stays exceeding 14 days.[16] The latter group's length of stay in the ICU averaged 24.5 days, the length of hospital stay averaged 57.9 days, and at 12 months, 44% of the survivors were still alive. The investigators found that the survivors had 12-month quality-of-life scores equal to those of other patients with shorter stays. The cost per year of life saved was Can$4350. One can compare the cost per year of life saved in this study with the cost of use of monoclonal antibodies in Gram-negative sepsis ($24,000) and conclude that the prolonged stay results are reasonable. However, the authors of the report pointed out that a strict analysis would have to include an assessment of the "opportunity costs" for prolonged stay; these costs would add amounts for interventions and programs that were not provided as a result of those that were.

Several strategies have been proposed to avoid the potential economic and social crisis that could result over the next 20 years of increased health care spending. If present trends continue, the cost to provide care for the elderly in 2020 will equal $25,000 per person per year, versus $9200 in 1995. If the current public and private shares of the cost remain unchanged, a large increase in taxes will be required. Several approaches can be used to reduce health care spending: 1) efforts can be made to reduce the increase in prices for resources that are used (e.g., by reducing physician payments), 2) efforts can be made to ensure that the same or more services are provided with fewer resources (i.e., by reducing nursing staffing levels), and 3) efforts can be made to slow the growth of services available to patients.[7]

The first two methods are unlikely to have additional sustained impact, because in many cases they have already been implemented and maximized by managed care over the last 10 years. The third method will require a concerted effort to ensure that ICU resources are allocated fairly. Table 3 lists principles for fair allocation of ICU resources from a recent position statement by the American Thoracic Society. The authors offered three goals that can be used to globally define the mission of the ICU. These goals are 1) to preserve meaningful human life by protecting and sustaining patients when they are threatened by an acute illness or injury, 2) to provide specialized rehabilitative care to patients as they begin to recover, and 3) to provide compassionate care to dying patients and their families, to ensure that suffering is alleviated. The 12 position statements that the authors used to describe the concept of fair resource allocation are summarized in Table 4. The 3rd and 11th statements are perhaps the most provocative because of their potential to affect the day-to-day practice of critical care medicine.

Table 3. Principles for fair allocation of intensive care unit (ICU) resources

Each individual's life is valuable and equally so.

Respect for patient autonomy, as represented by informed consent, is a central tenet for providing health care, including ICU care.

Enhancement of the patient's welfare is the primary duty of healthcare providers, by providing resources that meet an individual's medical needs and that the patient regards as beneficial.

ICU care, when medically appropriate, is an essential component of a basic package of healthcare services that should be available for all.

The duty of healthcare providers to benefit an individual patient has limits when doing so unfairly compromises the availability of resources needed by others.

Reproduced with permission from "Withholding and Withdrawing Life-Sustaining Therapy." *American Journal of Respiratory and Critical Care Medicine* 144:726–31, 1991.

The American Thoracic Society,[17] the Society of Critical Care Medicine,[18,19] and the American College of Chest Physicians[20] have all published position statements in which it is put forth that patients who are permanently unconscious should not be admitted to the ICU or have continued stay. Additionally, patients who have severe and permanent dementia, as well as those who meet criteria for brain death, should not receive intensive care.

The extent to which these position statements are adhered to in actual practice is not known. In a recent study, researchers analyzed the use in 1994 and 1995 of cardiopulmonary resuscitation (CPR) in ICU patients at 110 hospitals in 38 states.[21] Out of 74,502 admissions, there were 6303 deaths (8.5%). Excluding 393 patients with brain death, 23% of the patients received full intensive care and failed to respond to CPR, 22% received full intensive care without CPR, 10% had life support withheld (that is, the decision was made not to institute a medically appropriate and potentially beneficial therapy, with the knowledge that the patient would probably die without the intervention), and 38% had life support withdrawn. Despite the fact that about 70% of the patient population received some degree of limited care, there was enormous variability from facility to facility in the application of limits. The percentage of patients with do-not-resuscitate orders ranged from 0% to 83%, life support was withheld from 0% to 67%, and life support was withdrawn from 0% to 79%.

Conclusion

Recently, the Dutch parliament passed a measure that decriminalizes euthanasia. One commentator on the measure wrote, "The path to the death culture began when doctors learned to think like accountants. As the cost of socialized medicine in the Netherlands grew, doctors were lectured about the climbing cost of care. In many hospitals, signs were posted indicating how much old-age treatments cost taxpayers. The result was a growing 'social pressure' from doctors and others . . . which favors voluntary euthanasia."[22]

It would not be difficult to view the entire universe of critically ill patients in terms of payer class and mortality risk, to identify patients for whom aggressive care would not be predicted to be successful from either a clinical or financial standpoint. Steven Levitt,[23] a Harvard-educated economist and professor of economics at the University of Chicago, recently completed research that suggests that the reason the crime rate dropped sharply in the United States between 1992 and 1999 is that the legalization of abortion in the early 1970s reduced the number of potential future criminals. Similar reasoning would suggest that society could benefit from rationing care for certain kinds of critically ill patients even though rationing would result in the premature deaths of some people—the hope being that the conserved resources would be used to improve the overall health status of the population.

The fact remains that at some point in the process of rationing critical care, one human being or group of human beings needs to be able to look at another human being and make a decision to walk away, to discontinue, to shut down, to unplug. The question facing society and clinicians is, who will pull the trigger on Patient A? In trying to answer this question, it may be that, as suggested in one contemporary song, "life is a lesson—you'll learn it when you're through" (Limp Bizkit, "Take a Look Around").

Table 4. Summary of positions for fair allocation of
intensive care unit (ICU) resources

Access to ICU care requires that patients have sufficient medical need.

ICU care should provide the patient a certain degree of potential benefits. On the grounds of insufficient benefit to the patient, those who are permanently unconscious or who suffer from severe irreversible lack of cognitive function should generally be excluded from intensive care.

Whenever feasible, patients should give their informed consent for initiation and continuation of ICU care.

Patients should have equal access to ICU care regardless of their personal and behavioral characteristics.

ICU care should be equally available regardless of a patient's ability to pay.

When demand for ICU beds exceeds supply, medically appropriate patients should be admitted on a first-come, first-served basis. Because comparing degrees of benefit or need among patients competing for ICU care is morally problematic, as long as patients meet thresholds for medical need and benefit, they should be treated the same.

Access for marginally beneficial ICU care (i.e., care providing only minimal or a small incremental benefit) may be restricted on the basis of its limited benefit relative to cost. Decisions to restrict care on this basis should be made covertly by individual healthcare providers.

Prior to healthcare institutions limiting access to ICU care on the basis of limited benefit relative to cost, prerequisites for efficient use of healthcare resources, fair redistribution of savings, and public disclosure must be fulfilled.

Healthcare institutions and their providers should ensure availability of ICU beds by matching supply to medical need. Institutions should not initiate new programs that would increase demand for ICU care unless they provide additional ICU capacity and funding.

Once admitted to an ICU, qualified patients should generally receive all resources appropriate to meet their medical needs. Exceptions include if the scarce resource they need is already in use or if their consumption of a resource is so disproportionately great that its availability for others is endangered.

Healthcare institutions and their providers should limit access to ICU resources by means of explicit policies that are made known to patients and the public.

Patients and the public should be informed of financial incentives for limiting ICU care by physicians or healthcare institutions.

Reproduced with permission from "Withholding and Withdrawing Life-Sustaining Therapy." *American Journal of Respiratory and Critical Care Medicine* 144:726–31, 1991.

References

[1]O'Connor GT, Quinton HB, Traven ND, et al: Geographic variation in the treatment of acute myocardial infarction: the Cooperative Cardiovascular Project. JAMA 1999;281:627–33.

[2]Graboys TB: Coronary angiography: a long look at a short queue. JAMA 1999;282:184–5.

[3]McGrath PD, Wennberg DE, Dickens JD, et al: Relation between operator and hospital volume and outcomes following percutaneous coronary interventions in the era of the coronary stent. JAMA 2000;284:3139–44.

[4]Ware L, Matthay M: The acute respiratory distress syndrome. N Engl J Med 2000; 342:1334–49.

[5]Iglehart JK: The American health care system—Medicaid. N Engl J Med 1999;340:403–8.

[6]Gipe B: Financing critical care medicine in 2010. New Horiz 1999;7:184–97.

[7]McClellan M, Skinner J: Medicare reform: who pays and who benefits? Health Aff (Millwood) 1999;18:48–62.

[8]Iglehart JK: The American health care system—Medicare. N Engl J Med 1999;340:327–32.

[9]2000 tax table. Available at: http://www.irs.gov/ind_info/tax_tables/index.html. Accessed October 28, 2001.

[10]120 SCt 2143 (2000).

[11]Bloche MG, Jacobson PD: The Supreme Court and bedside rationing. JAMA 2000; 284:2776–9.

[12]Kralover P, Reczynski S: Profile of U.S. hospitals. Hosp Health Netw 2001;75:51–9.

[13]The American Hospital Association letter to Congress, August 5, 2000. Available at: http://www.aha.org/ar/advocacy/hsp-leadership-letter.asp. Accessed April 25, 2001.

[14]Page L: One in 10 California HMO practices are predicted to fail in 1999. AMNews. September 20, 1999.

[15]Singer PA, Martin DK, Kelner M: Quality end-of-life care: patients' perspectives. JAMA 1999;281:163–8.

[16]Heyland DK, Konopad E, Noseworthy TW, et al: Is it "worthwhile" to continue treating patients with a prolonged stay (>14 days) in the ICU? An economic evaluation. Chest 1998;114:192–8.

[17]Withholding and withdrawing life-sustaining therapy. This Official Statement of the American Thoracic Society was adopted by the ATS Board of Directors, March 1991. Am J Respir Crit Care Med 1991;144:726–31.

[18]Society of Critical Care Medicine Ethics Committee. Consensus statement on the triage of critically ill patients. JAMA 1994;271:1200–3.

[19]Consensus report on the ethics of foregoing life-sustaining treatments in the critically ill. Task Force on Ethics of the Society of Critical Care Medicine. Crit Care Med 1990;18:1435–9.

[20]Ethical and moral guidelines for the initiation, continuation, and withdrawal of intensive care. American College of Chest Physicians/Society of Critical Care Medicine Consensus Panel. Chest 1990;97:949–58.

[21]Prendergast TJ, Claessens MT, Luce JM: A national survey of end-of-life care for critically ill patients. Am J Respir Crit Care Med 1998;158:1163–7.

[22]Miniter R: The Dutch way of death. Wall Street Journal. April 25, 2001.

[23]Donohue JD, Levitt S: The impact of legalized abortion on crime. Quarterly Journal of Economics. 2001;116;379–420.

Globalization of Critical Care

John W. Hoyt, MD

I have been asked to review the clinical comments made about Patient A by critical care physicians from South Africa, Canada, Australia, the United Kingdom, India, New Zealand, the Netherlands, Russia, Hong Kong, Israel, and the United States. It is remarkable that such a task as this book was undertaken. Here, physicians from 11 countries, writing in English, the common language of science and medicine, share their thoughts on the prognosis and treatment of a 57-year-old man who had a cardiac arrest during cardiac catheterization.

There is only one way to explain the birth of this book. That is CCM-L (http://ccm-1.med.edu; an electronic bulletin board that is devoted to critical care medicine) and Dr. David Crippen, one of the book's editors. An avowed nonconformist and refugee from the 1960s, Dr. Crippen has connected intensive care unit (ICU) physicians from around the world by means of the Internet. He has single-handedly, without commercial sponsorship, woven a network of international intensivists. Nothing like this has ever occurred before. All readers of this book are being treated to a unique experience.

As a colleague, friend, and admirer of Dr. Crippen's for the last 14 years, I would like to analyze the 11 responses to Patient A not in terms of medical treatment but in terms of what Dr. Crippen has accomplished by creating CCM-L. The responses of the 11 physicians reviewing the treatment of this patient are in fact quite similar. One of the major differences relates to the availability of resources. A major similarity is the "whole patient" response by the intensivists.

I will cover the issues of physician duty, management of resources, the concept of the therapeutic trial, the role of the intensivist, and the future of critical care, with particular focus on the changing picture of critical care in the United States. All of these are addressed in the 11 responses to Patient A. As might be expected, I will of course give an American viewpoint on these issues, but I will also attempt to identify some themes that cross many cultures and approaches to the delivery of health care.

Duty

The father of medicine is the great Greek physician Hippocrates. From his writings has grown the code of professional ethics that guides the practice of medicine in many countries, particularly in the Western world. This is nicely pointed out by Dr. van der Spoel from the Netherlands in his discussion of Patient A's case. He reminds readers that Hippocrates would call physicians to treat every patient who seeks their help, to respect the patient, to act in the best interest of the patient, and to do no harm. He further states that treating every patient does not mean applying every conceivable technology to every patient. It is the duty of the intensivist to determine which patients will likely respond to treatment and benefit from intensive care and to focus "curing" resources on these patients. Likewise, it is appropriate for the intensivist to identify patients who will not recover and to focus "caring" or palliative resources on these patients.

How does one translate this across many countries and cultures? For me, the big issue is availability of resources. How does one deal with the issue of duty to patients in the Hippocratic sense when there is great knowledge of medical care on the part of the intensivist and at the same time great limitation of resources? I was struck by the comments of Dr. Burrows from South Africa. He works in a 750-bed hospital that has only 8 ICU beds. He cares for 500 patients a year. Every day he must make difficult decisions about whom he will treat and whom he will comfort. In the case of Patient A, he responds that the probability of survival is low in comparison with that for other more needy patients. Thus he would reject making a treatment commitment to this patient.

As one might expect, this is very difficult for an American physician to swallow. In the United States, $1.2 trillion (14% of the gross domestic product) is spent on health care each year, and rarely if ever are American intensivists forced to make decisions about whom they will treat on the basis of availability of resources. This is not to say that the United States is without rationing. Millions of American patients are without health insurance and in the same category as Patient A. These patients have real trouble managing their ambulatory health care needs. However, if they become critically ill, they can easily enter the health care system and end up in the ICU, there to receive thousands of dollars of treatment per day.

Thus when Dr. Burrows suggests that he would not admit this patient to the ICU, I recoil in my uniquely American way. But on further contemplation, I can see that Dr. Burrows is employing triage and serving patients with the best chance of survival, using the resources at his fingertips. Dr. Batchelor from the United Kingdom makes very similar comments. She has limited resources compared with physicians in other countries, and she must think first about whom she can help before she launches into treating a patient and consuming precious resources that might be needed by patients more likely to have favorable outcomes.

In the United States, the physician who has spoken most eloquently about professional duty is Dr. Edmund D. Pellegrino, a clinician and ethicist at Georgetown University. In his book *Helping and Healing* (cowritten with David C. Thomasma), he wrote, "Treatment of the ill requires sensitivity to patient values, and care for persons rather than for political and economic abstractions. Medical decisions must fuse the good of the patient with the scientifically correct decision. Thus medicine invariably turns on a moral option—as a fusion of technology and morality in which the regulating element is what ought to be done, not only what can be done."[1]

Management of Resources

In the case of Patient A, what is the moral thing to do? I think this book points to a new understanding of the phrase "what ought to be done." In many ways, the job description of the intensivist is something unimagined by Hippocrates. Intensivists have split obligations. They have a duty to use their resources in as scientifically sound a way as possible while exercising principles of triage and rationing so that patients most likely to survive will receive what they need to survive. Intensivists also have a duty to patients already in the ICU and to future patients who might survive—a duty to hold back resources from those with a poor prognosis. Those resources are "banked," saved for those whom intensivists know they can help.

Critical care physicians in the United States have rarely if ever had to make such day-to-day triage decisions. A recent book coedited by Dr. George D. Lundberg, former editor of the *Journal of the American Medical Association,* explores the unique American problem. In that book, entitled *Severed Trust,*[2] the case is made that American physicians use medical resources based on the principle of "what they can" use rather than on what "they ought" to use. Thus Americans spend more than $1.2 trillion on health care annually. This is clearly not the moral or right thing for physicians to do in the exercise of their professional duty to patients.

It seems to me that in the context of the current book, the moral or right thing for the intensivist to do is to determine what ought to be done for Patient A in the light of available resources, scientifically sound treatment principles, and the need of the patient. Thus in South Africa, Patient A does not get an ICU bed, whereas in the United States, he gets the full technology. Both are right decisions in those countries. But the burden on Dr.

Chalfin in the United States is not to get caught up in what can be done but instead to determine, based on conversation with the family and the analysis of evidence-based medicine, what ought to be done. Dr. Chalfin has uniquely unlimited resources and the pressure to "do everything." As a good intensivist, he has learned to withstand that pressure and apply sensible scientific principles in the treatment of patients with life-threatening illnesses.

For American intensivists, there are two potential perversions of intensive care that exist uniquely in a system with unlimited funds. On the one hand, the American intensivist can easily "do everything" and not be viewed by his colleagues as deviating from standard American medical practice. Likewise, the American intensivist can also withhold treatment on the basis of some personal agenda of saving money for a nebulous cause. Money saved with the idea that it might be transferred to vaccination programs for children or ambulatory care for the uninsured will never make it to those programs in different sites in the United States. There is no way that $10,000 I might save in an ICU in Pittsburgh will be funneled to a poor neighborhood in Chicago for the care of needy children. Thus, I should not withhold potentially helpful treatment from an ICU patient in the name of some higher cause. I must fall back on the guiding principles of Dr. Pellegrino—namely, to do what is scientifically sound and medically appropriate for each patient in the ICU. If reallocation of resources in the United States ever occurs, it needs to be done with some community agreement on how Americans will spend their health care dollars.

Therapeutic Trial

Dr. Streat from New Zealand brings up an important consideration for those countries with generous resources. He would agree to admit this patient to the ICU, but "with reservations," while he was determining the central nervous system status of the patient and the patient's ability to recover from the cardiac arrest. Clearly, even very seasoned intensivists, such as Dr. Streat, recognize their inability to predict outcome accurately in many situations. I would call this an ICU admission for a therapeutic trial. Basically, I need a few days (5–7 days) of aggressive treatment to evaluate the likely outcome for this type of patient. I agree with Dr. Streat that the major issue is the degree of neurological damage.

Historically, there has been a hesitancy among American physicians working in the ICU to conduct a therapeutic trial. A not-infrequent teaching is that a physician should never intubate a patient with advanced chronic obstructive lung disease, because he or she will never get off the ventilator. I think that is foolish. It is perfectly acceptable to withdraw life support and make a patient comfortable while end-stage chronic obstructive pulmonary disease takes the life of the patient if the therapeutic trial fails. It is important to address this issue and communicate these plans to the family from the beginning. Relatives must know that a therapeutic trial is not an open door to unending life support when there is no hope of recovery. The family must know in some detail how the physician will deal with end-of-life care if the patient fails to improve and respond to treatment. Most families, but not all, will share in this decision making with the physician.

Role of the Intensivist

Credit also goes to Dr. Streat for bringing up the issue of the intensivist versus the "single organ doctor" (e.g., pulmonologist, cardiologist, or nephrologist). This is not a criticism of these important specialists, who are part of the team managing a patient with a life-threatening illness but who tend not to manage the whole patient. The evolution of medical specialists in much of Europe and all of Australia and New Zealand differed from that in the United States. From the beginning, intensivists managing whole patients have been the predominant model in Europe, Australia, and New Zealand. The United States instead developed a powerful culture of organ-specific specialization. Such specialization has led to a fragmentation of the care of critically ill patients, lengthening ICU stays and increasing the cost of care. Pronovost et al[3] recently showed clearly that length of stay is shortened and mortality is reduced threefold when an intensivist team rounds daily on ICU patients and coordinates all aspects of care.

Critical Care in the United States

Only 10% of ICUs in the United States have full-time intensivists coordinating care. In 90% of situations, mostly in urban, suburban, and rural community hospitals, care is delivered using the fragmented, organ-specialty approach just described. An Institute of Medicine report suggests that medical errors in American hospitals take the lives of 100,000 patients annually.[4] The article by Pronovost et al[3] suggests that many of these lives, up to 58,000 per year, could be lives of patients in the ICU. A coalition of American businesses called the Leapfrog Group[5] is calling for sweeping changes in American medicine. The coalition wants physician orders entered into computer databases, complicated surgeries done only in institutions with high volumes of surgeries, and all ICUs managed by full-time intensivists. These businesses intend to spend their dollars only in ICUs that can meet their standards. The coalition, along with the follow-up report on quality care by the Institute of Medicine,[6] may drive ICUs in the United

States to assume the full-time intensivist model. Data indicate that this will save thousands of lives and millions, if not billions, of dollars each year.

I suspect that these changes in American critical care will take 10–20 years to accomplish. The changes will be worth it. Currently, if Patient A is admitted to one of the urban hospitals in America without an intensivist coordinating care, there will be a neurologist taking care of the concern over central nervous system damage from the cardiac arrest, a cardiologist taking care of the hypotension and cardiac output, and a nephrologist taking care of the renal failure. The three specialists will not commonly speak to each other and will leave illegible notes (their only means of communication) in the chart. There will be no physician or intensivist to coordinate care, and the application of technology will go on for days and days. The description by Dr. Chalfin of how this patient would be managed in the United States is misleading. He describes care given in 10% of the ICUs in the United States. Dr. Crippen looked for someone to speak for the 90% of American ICUs without an intensivist, but he could not find anyone in charge.

References

[1]Pellegrino ED, Thomasma DC: Helping and Healing: Religious Commitment in Health Care. Translated. Washington, DC: Georgetown University Press, 1997, p. 5.
[2]Lundberg GD, Stacey J: Severed Trust: Why American Medicine Hasn't Been Fixed. New York, NY: Basic Books, 2001.
[3]Pronovost PJ, Jenckes MW, Dorman T, et al: Organizational characteristics of intensive care units related to outcomes of abdominal aortic surgery. JAMA 281:1310–7.
[4]Kohn LT, Corrigan JM, Donaldson MS (eds): To Err Is Human. Washington, DC: National Academy Press, 2000.
[5]Leapfrog Group Web site. Available at: http://www.leapfroggroup.org. Accessed October 15, 2001.
[6]Committee on Quality Health Care in America, Institute of Medicine: Crossing the Quality Chasm: A New Health System for the 21st Century. Washington, DC: National Academy Press, 2001.

A Multilevel Examination of a Critically Ill Patient

Jack K. Kilcullen, MD, JD, MPH

(special thanks to Nancy Dubler, LLB,
and staff of the Montefiore Medical Center Department of Bioethics)

Should Patient A Be Treated?

Critical care medicine carries with it the challenge that there be no edge too far from which a life cannot be pulled back to safety. Lives all but lost are routinely saved through mechanical ventilation, fluid resuscitation, and use of inotropic and vasopressor agents and antibiotics—all administered in a tightly monitored setting. Technology reaches deep into the physical frame, often without penetrating the skin, to track changes in vascular forces, shifts in chemical concentrations, and disruptions of anatomy. International research explores physiology under the most extreme of stresses to bring new insights to the intensive care bedside.

Yet a 10-bed intensive care unit (ICU) still has only 10 beds, no matter how many resources benefit the occupant of each one. (How many resources indeed reach each bed is itself a subtler but no less significant issue.) Whereas regular inpatient services may always have room for one more, for many ICUs there is simply no such thing as an empty bed. The line at the door is not only constant but constantly changing, given that the one next in line may get bumped at the last minute by someone deemed more in need. The line for the last bed is longer still, for it now includes not only real patients but the hypothetical patient always sicker than those at hand, the patient who may show up just when the bed is being assigned.

For the physician in the ICU, the decision to admit is a tangle of medical, monetary, and moral factors for which no international consensus exists. A relatively young man, healthy despite his occult atherosclerosis, Patient A is caught in a cascade of complications that seem guaranteed to ensue when a high-tech intervention is attempted in an otherwise low-tech arena, where single-organ care resulted in multiple organ failure. He presents in extremis, with possibly two kinds of shock and with oxygenation deeply impaired, and is unable to clear his body of toxins and fluid. His level of consciousness is seemingly negligible.

The fate of Patient A, who seems like the ideal ICU patient, varies considerably depending on the passport in his pocket:

- In the Netherlands, full resuscitation and treatment would begin immediately, with hope for signs of full recovery over the next 3 days.
- In New Zealand, admission to the ICU would be resisted because of his profound neurological injury; in the United Kingdom, in addition, initial resuscitation would have to have commenced prior to transfer.
- In Israel, treatment would be undertaken, but given physician staffing limitations, the patient's survival would be highly problematic.
- In South Africa, his poor overall prognosis, given the profound paucity of hospital resources, would preclude any treatment whatsoever.
- In Canada, the treatment is similar to the United States except for more of a "take a number for better service" entry scheme to health services.

The critical care physician is trained to examine each threat, prioritize it, and attack it in a swift and systematic fashion. In Australia, for instance, invasive and noninvasive monitoring of cardiac output would be started to establish the nature of his poor perfusion. Inotropic agents to improve the heart's performance would be given, and fluids would be added or removed as needed to correct his volume status. The ventilator would be manipulated to rectify the ventilation/perfusion ratio and reduce the required FIO_2. Should renal failure persist, continuous hemofiltration would be used to help remove excess fluid and cleanse the blood. "Therapy would not be stopped for at least 3 days, unless signs of brain injury appeared clinically," writes Dr. Fisher from Australia.

The patient's depressed consciousness at the outset would seemingly not deter the Australians from their plan of action. Similarly, in Hong Kong, the existence of additional funds would not alter the plan of care but would only result in there being additional staff to carry it out. The patient's presenting neurological injury does not merit great concern: "Intravenous infusions of morphine and midazolam would be titrated to achieve analgesia and comfort. These infusions would then be intermittently discontinued to assess neurological status." In the Netherlands, initial resuscitation would take priority; only on day 3 would neurological status be seriously studied.

Yet the medical and the moral collide in the minds of those contributors who consider his neurological status of threshold concern and who begin by asking whether he will survive the war even if his physician wins the immediate battle. Despite the sedation he might have received, there is ample indication that his hypoxemia is such that he has only enough viable neuroanatomy to maintain basic physiological functions. The persistent vegetative state may well be the best this patient can achieve, and if so, there are physicians who are openly questioning whether this justifies the use of all the resources required. For most of those who debate the question, resource limitations are not the issue, at least officially. That is, they would not treat past a certain point, if at all, because the patient will not recover neurologically, even if resources are unlimited. In the presence of medical futility, they argue, there is a moral obligation not to treat.

Compassionate as this sounds from those trained to "do everything," the thorniness of the issues it raises may lead one to question whether this approach may actually be self-serving. How does anyone truly know this patient's potential for recovery, especially at the initial encounter? What are the odds, and with what certainty are they known? What must the odds be? What lies behind that judgment? Are there subtle influences of prejudice, or competing demands elsewhere in the ICU at that moment? Is the clinician who is dealing with the case—one requiring quick and complex decisions—physically exhausted? And who, if anyone, may be allowed to speak for the patient? Are family members arguing not just that everything be done but that the patient would want everything done, that he has children who depend on him? Medical futility is not merely a clinical assessment; it is a judgment that triggers the withdrawal of life-sustaining measures. When physicians play God, as only ICU physicians do as a matter of course, they exercise immense power unmatched outside the judicial system and with hardly a whisper of the safeguards that characterize that system. To the family who protests, it can amount to an execution of a death sentence with little trial and no right of appeal.

Although the decision not to treat appears settled in some countries, according to certain contributors, its relevance to Patient A remains bitterly contested, particularly in the United States. Dr. Streat writes that in New Zealand, the patient would not reach the ICU given his neurological state, unless there was some ambiguity in the record to suggest that sedation might be at work. Only then would admission to the ICU be allowed, and only on a conditional basis, which has been formalized as follows:

> Under such circumstances, we might admit the patient to the ICU to determine the neurological prognosis and provide supportive care until that determination could be made. This type

of admission is known as an admission with reservations. It represents the first level of three stages of limitation of intensive therapies (reservations, specific limitations, and withdrawal are the three stages) that are an integral part of the way we practice. Admitting a patient with reservations acts as a signal that intensive therapies may be limited or withdrawn if the patient does not make good progress. In this situation, intensive therapies (including, for example, correction of hypoxia, correction of hypotension, and clearing of residual sedation by dialysis) might be administered for 48 hours, pending an assessment of neurological status and reversibility of multiple organ failure. The assessment might include various neurological tests (magnetic resonance imaging, electroencephalography, somatosensory evoked potential testing) in addition to serial neurological examinations. Should this assessment show that severe HIE [hypoxic-ischemic encephalopathy] was present, intensive therapies would be withdrawn by the intensivists in the context of consensus among any other treating physicians and the patient's family.

If the record showed that no sedation had been given, and therefore sedation was not the reason for the patient's depressed consciousness, the intensivist would document his denial of admission by his assessment of the patient's poor prognosis:

The patient's severe multiple organ failure is multifactorial, including aspiration and cardiogenic shock post-CPR [cardiopulmonary resuscitation], and he may now have early nosocomial pneumonia. This syndrome alone would carry a high mortality, especially in the absence of mechanically reversible cardiac dysfunction. I suggest that you discuss this situation fully and frankly with the patient's family and advise the family that intensive therapies be withdrawn and a comfort care plan be instituted. We would be happy to give further advice on request.

Dr. Streat's facility has only "14 beds capable of supporting mechanical ventilation," but he states, "We are able in emergency situations to take more patients, and we would not deny a clinically suitable and appropriate patient admission solely on the grounds of resource constraint."

Dr. Batchelor from the United Kingdom makes similar comments:

As presented, Patient A has multiple organ failure with respiratory, renal, cardiovascular, hepatic, and neurological failure. My major concern at this stage would be whether this man would respond neurologically to salvage treatment. All inter-ICU transfers should be made on a consultant-to-consultant referral basis. Before accepting this patient for transfer, I would want to know what sedation he had received, if any, and what his current best responses were. At 3 days post–hypoxic-ischemic event, if the patient has abnormal brain stem responses, absent verbal response, absent withdrawal to painful stimuli, and a significantly increased serum creatinine level, he has a very poor chance of survival with or without severe disability. In addition to his original insult, this patient appears to have had a continuing insult; this normally hypertensive man has hypotension. If I were not satisfied with the responses, I would get in my car and go look at the patient before agreeing to his transfer. Patients can be "dumped" on me only if I agree; in the United Kingdom, hospitals do not accept other hospitals' patients—doctors do.

Dr. Kapadia from India, where there is no pressure of cost constraints, yet where the ICU is "invariably full," writes, "What would I do on arrival of the patient to the ICU? First I would decide if there was a realistic chance of brain recovery. Presuming that to be the case, I would proceed to manage the etiological events as well as correct the deranged physiology." One would assume that in the absence of neurological viability, such management would not take place.

By contrast, in the Netherlands, all efforts to resuscitate the patient would be prioritized and undertaken. Last on the list is to

tell the family that the prognosis was grim, especially in terms of cerebral function. I would explain that we were trying to improve the patient's general condition and that maybe with optimizing of his general function, his cerebral function would improve. If, however, his cerebral condition were not to improve, and especially if somato-sensory evoked potentials were absent, all therapy would be stopped, because he would never regain consciousness.

The physician's obligation to provide what he or she considers to be futile care has been vigorously debated over the past 20 years in the United States. Definitions of the word *futility* vary. According to Schneiderman and colleagues,[1] a treatment has to have more than a physiological effect; it has to have a broader benefit for the patient beyond that which "merely preserves permanent consciousness or . . . fails to end a patient's total dependence on intensive medical care." Attempts to offer a quantitative basis for the threshold of futility have foundered because of 1) lack of empiric evidence (e.g., models such as the Acute Physiology and Chronic Health Evaluation system are limited by their applicability only to groups), 2) the arbitrariness of choosing a percentage of success that an intervention must meet (must it be 20% likely, or 5%?) and 3) the goal of the treatment itself, such as keeping a patient alive to see family members again.

These subjective questions of how much of life is still worth living challenge the roles physicians have assumed in making them. Lantos et al[2] argued that only patients could meaningfully address this. The challenge to this position is that the physician becomes merely the servant of the patient and the family, rather than a moral agent with professional integrity on whom that patient and the patient's family have relied for objectivity and expertise. Good communication can prevent conflicts between individual families and physicians even when there remains no consensus in society at large. However, in many American ICUs, as Dr. Chalfin from the United States points out, there simply is no intensivist in charge of a patient's care:

> Many scenarios for the delivery of critical care services exist, yet the common feature of most is the presence of multiple consultants called on behalf of the primary care physician or the attending of record, each one addressing his or her area of expertise. In Patient A's case, the cardiologist might be the person who inserts the pulmonary artery catheter and could even serve as the one who decides among the various antiarrhythmics, inotropes, and vasopressors. A pulmonary specialist would be called to manage the ventilator and to consult about the ARDS [acute respiratory distress syndrome] and aspiration. An infectious disease physician might also be involved, especially if the patient continued to exhibit leukocytosis and manifest signs of sepsis. In addition, a nephrologist would be asked to provide input regarding the azotemia and the decreased urinary output. It is also likely that a hematology consultation would be requested, given the patient's coagulopathy, and a gastroenterologist and/or liver specialist might be solicited for advice as well, in view of the transaminitis. It is important to recognize that although consultants usually attempt to contact the physician of record and keep him or her informed of their impressions and actions, they often work independently of one another in an episodic fashion.
>
> With respect to involvement by a critical care practitioner, the pulmonary physician will often have expertise and perhaps even board certification in critical care; however, in all too many cases, he or she focuses only on the respiratory system and defers other problems to the cadre of other consultants.

This fragmentation leads not only to a lack of organizational clarity with regard to the treatment plan, but to inconsistent messages to the family concerning the very question of futility—with pulmonologists, anesthesiologists, and surgeons traditionally differing in how "realistic" or "optimistic" their opinions can sound. Procedural safeguards through informal consultation via neutral parties are an important tool to bring physicians a step back from their decisions, to give time for families to participate in the decision-making process. Multidisciplinary bodies, such as the Bioethics Consultation Service at Montefiore Medical Center, employ techniques of conflict resolution to help parties reestablish the trust lost in the tragedy of the patient's illness.

Mediation serves to give balance and legitimacy to both medical and family points of view. This can serve to resolve conflicts due largely to misunderstanding or mistrust. The fact that there are powerful tools at physicians' disposal does not mean that physicians have unbridled freedom in using them. Similarly, the right to high-quality service as a health care consumer does not come with the guarantee of a happy outcome. The hope is that better communication between patients' families and physicians, directly or with the help of third parties, can reconcile their divergent expectations.

In the end, however, physicians' exclusive role in deciding if and when to withdraw care remains sharply limited by judicial decision in the United States, where courts have almost universally sided with the family and against the hospital on the question of withdrawing treatment. Indeed, even in the absence of advance directives, the family, when united, is given great deference when the "benefit" of medical interventions to which a patient is entitled is being defined. In *Barber v Superior Court,*[3] criminal charges were brought against two physicians who, at the family's bequest, stopped nasogastric feeding and intravenous hydration in their patient, who had experienced profound ischemic encephalopathy during a routine surgical procedure. The family had sought to end "heroic measures," which included mechanical ventilation, although the patient continued to breathe spontaneously. When nutrition was similarly withdrawn, a nurse alerted the local district attorney, who began proceedings. After 2 years, the court concluded that nutrition was a "medical procedure," the continuation of which depended on the weighing of benefits and burdens. When the hoped-for benefits are outweighed, the measures can be withdrawn.

Yet when the family similarly insists on heroic measures, no demonstration of futility is sufficient to overcome this insistence. Two celebrated cases involve mechanical ventilation. In Minnesota, a probate court considered the fate of Helga Wanglie, an 86-year-old woman who developed respiratory failure secondary to nosocomial pneumonia following a successful repair of a fractured hip. After many months, a period punctuated by multiple attempts at weaning and an episode of resuscitation from a cardiopulmonary arrest that left her with profound brain injury, the treating hospital sought to terminate mechanical ventilation out of the belief that both her dependence and her susceptibility to infection made further ventilation futile. Her family was deeply religious, and although the husband acknowledged the depth of her deterioration and that her own views were unknown, he said that "we hope for the best." She died while still receiving mechanical ventilation, 3 days after the court ruled in her husband's favor.

In the case *In re Baby K,*[4] the United States Court of Appeals for the Fourth Circuit interpreted the Emergency Medical Treatment and Active Labor Act,[5] which requires hospitals to provide appropriate emergency care, as upholding the right of a mother to insist on continued mechanical ventilation for an anencephalic infant. This decision was reached over the objections of pediatric specialists, who described Baby K as lacking a cerebral cortex as well as part of her skull and scalp; she could not see, think, feel, or interact with the world around her and thus was described as permanently unconscious, for which no treatment exists. They articulated the medical standard of care that mechanical ventilation not be provided to such an impaired infant. Commentators have argued in support of the mother, who described herself as deeply religious; they have said that the belief in the sanctity of life overrides judgments made by physicians who consider medically futile those procedures that would fail to restore a certain quality of life.

Philosopher Helga Kuhse discussed the unqualified "sanctity-of-life principle": "It is absolutely prohibited either intentionally to kill a patient or intentionally to let a patient die, and to base decisions relating to the prolongation or shortening of human life on considerations of its quality or kind."[6] Kuhse, citing both Jewish and Christian literature, concluded that *sanctity* refers to the infinite value of every fraction of human life. The battle is joined by an array of disparate groups, including fundamentalist Christians, orthodox Jews (as well as those mindful of the treatment of Jews and others at the hands of the Nazis), and advocates for people with disabilities. Wolf Wolfensberger, one such advocate, proposed "an unequivocal position on the value of all human life, including the lives of impaired people of all ages at any stage of life, at any level of capacity, and of any degree of moral goodness. Bodies that claim to represent, and to advocate for, impaired people are called upon to uphold a coherent position on the sanctity of all human life." He condemned the "dishonest bioethics culture" as "death-making."[7]

In stark contrast, families elsewhere in the world possess no such veto power. In the United Kingdom, for instance,

> the family would be informed that the outlook was guarded and there was still a significant probability that he would die. All we would be able to do is provide the appropriate conditions for him to get better. We would provide all treatment possible at the moment and continuously review the situation. If it became clear that he was not responding to treatment or indeed was deteriorating, we would tell the family and discuss treatment withdrawal. Treatment withdrawal is a medical decision made by a group of doctors and nurses. We do not ask a patient's relatives to make these decisions; we merely want them to understand and agree with our decision.

Dr. van der Spoel from the Netherlands describes much-heralded court decisions in cases involving administration of extraordinary care to a brain-injured infant and to a terminally ill elderly father. The physicians were permitted to act according to their medical judgment and without feeling compelled to "do everything" when there was nothing left to do.

In the United States, the balance of power between physicians and patients and their families has not remained static. However, what has perhaps begun to push aside this tug-of-war is an evolution in the public's understanding of the issue—an understanding that life does indeed come to an end and that physicians have a vital if still rarely exercised role in easing the pain and fear of the patient in his or her closing days. The maturation of the hospice movement and the establishment of expertise in palliative care mean the existence of new tools, and obviously new hope that physicians, patients, and families will recognize that they stand on common ground.

Thus, although critical care physicians have similar training around the world, their concepts of patient viability and patient autonomy do not translate so neatly, resulting in drastically different courses of action.

How Much Is There to Spend?

Apart from moral obligations, money matters deeply. Among the international consultants for whom resources are plentiful, what they would do and what they would do if they had unlimited resources and authority are the same. In South Africa, by contrast, there is nothing to do, because the patient's multiplicity of problems means that attempts to save him would very visibly and immediately deprive others of help who had more hope.

Inpatient mortality in South Africa is often 40%, in part reflecting the acuity of the conditions of those who finally make it to the hospital, in part reflecting the lack of resources along every mile they traveled. A world of unlimited resources was so abstract to Dr. Burrows from South Africa that he found it absurd to put his approach in that situation into words.

What is also intriguing is the degree of sensitivity physicians around the world have to the logistical constraints on the care they provide. Whereas Dr. Kapadia from India considered the cost of care to be a matter for the bean counters and business people ("it is up to management to balance the books"), Dr. Batchelor from the United Kingdom had such detailed knowledge of resource restraints that she found the scenario hard to imagine: How is it that this patient underwent angioplasty in the first place, given that fewer than 5 of the 17 hospitals who might have first treated him have the resources to resort to angioplasty to treat his myocardial infarction? The logistical challenge of traveling by helicopter for the angioplasty is all but insurmountable, because the scarce hospital helicopters are reserved for those yet to reach the hospital. Dr. Batchelor worried about the traffic and the difficulties that the team of paramedics assigned to manage the patient in the helicopter would face to get a ride back to their own facility.

Moreover, a patient's probability of success must be weighed against real and potential competitors for an ICU bed, when resource limitations take the form of bed limits. In South Africa, for example, "the prognosis is grim, and the probability of death under these circumstances is extremely high. Thus a choice must necessarily be made among patients. If this patient were to be offered the ICU bed, there is every likelihood that others with a better chance of survival would be denied treatment." In the United Kingdom, acceptance of the patient would hinge on his odds for dramatic improvement before transfer, because unlike in India, hospital administrators do not leave physicians free to accept whomever they wish:

> I would insist that he be appropriately resuscitated before transfer, to include administration of fluids, inotropes, and more appropriate ventilation. If his condition could not be optimized before transfer, I would refuse to accept him. If necessary, I would send out a senior trainee or consultant to supervise resuscitation and transfer; however, we are not funded for this. Interhospital transfers are audited for number, reason, and quality.

Who manages the resources in the ICU varies. In Russia, the choice of the patient's attending depends on the dominant organ system impaired: "Each patient in the intensive care unit . . . must be admitted by one of the clinical departments according to the leading syndrome. The attending physician (usually the chief of the department), not an intensivist, develops the general treatment plan and prognosis."

In many ICUs in the United States, where the patient's private attending controls the admission, the intensivist is but one of a number of consulting specialists. What this means is that control of the ICU as a precious resource is in no one's hands—or, rather, in the hands of the individual physician who managed to transfer his or her patient there. This physician is the one who decides when to relinquish the bed, and he or she therefore has an overriding moral as well as personal interest in that patient and not in the patients who are waiting for the bed.

What resources each bed has and whom each patient must compete against ultimately determine the intensity of care. In Israel,

> there is no 24-hour in-house attending, and it might not be possible to have a physician at the patient's bedside all the time. . . . only physicians take the hemodynamic profile. If the other patients in the ICU did not require constant physician attention, the patient would be managed according to plan. If another patient, perhaps with a better prognosis, needed similar attention, corners would be cut and the patient would probably die.

In many developing nations, there arises the question of whether ICUs should exist at all. Certainly, many preventive health interventions, funded by the amount spent on running an ICU for a week, are able to save many more lives. Even the routine care offered by the most modest of community hospitals seems wasteful compared with the work of those in water management, sanitation, and agricultural development. In fact, only in recent years has the World Health Organization (which has spent millions on nutrition programs for women in developing countries) recognized that primary school education for girls can have a profound impact in later years on infant mortality and family nutrition as these literate, better-informed girls become mothers. With so much to do, the question then becomes, how many doctors, let alone the tools at their disposal, can the world afford?

Of course, little in the area of resource allocation is truly global. Wealth is so lopsided that types as well as availability of ICUs vary. (Here at Montefiore Medical Center, we have the range, from general medical and general surgical to cardiac, pulmonary, and cardiothoracic.) There is also great disparity within countries. Dr. Kapadia from India writes, "In our hospital, medical care is rarely if ever withheld for lack of funds." Resource allocation is not just ethical and political, but also deeply cultural. In the

1980s, Canada followed Europe and dumped its market-driven system of health care financing and turned to a national plan, which, despite its limitations, remains a source of national pride. In the United States, the requisite sense of social responsibility remains a distinctly foreign notion, and Americans continue to reject any such public solution, even as dissatisfaction with the existing system deepens.

Yet despite that rejection, basic access to health care must exist. The President's Commission for the Study of Ethical Problems in Medicine and Biomedical and Behavioral Research established:

> In the United States, quality of opportunity is a widely accepted value that is refected throughout public policy. . . . In this view, health care is that which people need to maintain or restore normal functioning or to compensate for inability to function normally. Health is thus comparable in importance to education in determining the opportunity available to people to pursue life plans.
>
> . . . Although neither "everything needed" nor "everything beneficial" nor "everything that anyone else is getting" are defensible ways of understanding equitable access, the special nature of health care dictates that everyone have access to *some* level of care: enough care to achieve sufficient welfare, opportunity, information and evidence interpersonal concern to facilitate a reasonably full and satisfying life. . . .
>
> It is the Commission's view that the societal obligation to ensure equitable access for everyone may be best fulfilled in this country by a pluralistic approach that relies upon the coordinated contributions by both the private and public sectors.[8]

Yet if one assumes that health care resources are finite (indeed, what nation in the past 10 years has not been forced to make painful choices for its population?), critical care is the paradox: it exists as a product of a public health process, with each society choosing—through its own system of allocating health care resources—to designate 1% or 2% of a hospital's beds for its sickest patients. Yet those few members of the public entitled to those beds are selected under acute conditions and often on the basis of incomplete knowledge. The complexity of critical care and the public fears of critical illness leave people largely unaware of how physicians at the door of the ICU daily weigh the viability of a patient and the value of a life against the availability of a bed and the number of pulmonary artery catheter kits in the supply room. Will this be the patient who always looks 48 hours away from turning around, even after 2 weeks have passed?

In Patient A's case, any deliberating at the door of the ICU may mean his death. For the intensivist first on the scene, training and instinct may remove the sensation of choice at all. Fluids will be administered, vasopressor therapy begun, and the ventilator adjusted so that time can be gained to decide what to do next. What the contributors have given the readers of this book is only part of the story. The choices a society makes regarding how much of its wealth it devotes to the health of its members are made not only by physicians but by administrators and politicians and, most of all, by all persons as they act each day in ways that will either impair or improve their own health and thus increase or reduce the costs that society must ultimately bear.

References

[1]Schneiderman LF, Jecker NS, Jonsen AR: Medical futility: its meaning and ethical implications. Ann Intern Med 1990;112:949–54.

[2]Lantos JD, Singer PA, Walker RM, et al: The illusion of futility in clinical practice. Am J Med 1989;87:81–4.

[3]195 Cal Rptr 484, 489 (Ct App 1983).

[4]832 F Supp 1022 (ED Va 1993), *aff'd,* 16 F3d 590 (4th Cir), *cert denied,* 115 SCt 91 (1994).

[5]542 USC §1395.

[6]Kuhse H. Quoted by Post SG: Baby K: medical futility and the free exercise of religion. J Law Med Ethics 1995;23:20–6.

[7]Wolfensberger W. Quoted by Post SG: Baby K: medical futility and the free exercise of religion. J Law Med Ethics 1995;23:20–6.

[8]The President's Commission for the Study of Ethical Problems in Medicine and Biomedical and Behavioral Research: An Ethical Framework for Access to Health Care. Quoted by Arras JD, Steinbock B: Ethical Issues in Modern Medicine. 5th ed. Mountain View, CA: Mayfield, 1999.

Patient B

The Decision-Making Process

Rolando Berger, MD

Patient B clearly exemplifies a dilemma often faced by critical care practitioners everywhere. The 11 critical care physicians representing 11 countries and all 5 populated continents agree that aggressive intensive care in this context would be futile. There is no real debate among them about the very small chance that this patient could survive his current illness, and certainly none about the fact that his quality of life after this episode, if by some miracle he were to survive for a few additional months or years, would be as dismal as before and in all likelihood significantly worse. However, although all 11 physicians believe this quite strongly, only a few of them state unequivocally that they would not provide this level of care in any case, regardless of the family's request. Clearly a problem exists at the level of implementation. Those who might end up providing this care would do so because social-legal pressures compel them, despite their own judgment that such efforts are futile. None of the physicians indicate feeling ethically compelled to provide care that they are convinced is medically futile.

In one form or another, several of the physicians analyzing this case point out that an improved communication process with intensive care unit (ICU) patients and their families should obviate this type of problem, and one physician goes so far as to indicate that within his own ICU practice, he perceives persistence of unreasonable requests almost as a personal failure in this endeavor. Indeed, a "procedural approach" that involves frank communication between health care personnel and the patient and his or her family is almost universally proposed as the first and most useful step in resolving conflicts about futility.[1]

It is probably correct to assume that many (most?) "unreasonable" requests for futile care derive from an incomplete understanding of the limitations of certain treatment modalities, the irreversible nature of a given disease process, and/or the true nature of the outcome likely to be obtained and what would be involved in trying to achieve it. These cases can be managed with relative ease through a procedural approach, either formal or informal, which stresses the importance of frank, respectful, and honest communication between health providers and their patients and families.[2] However, stopping at this recommendation is really nothing more than avoiding the real issue. The problem lies not here but with cases in which the request for continuous care that is deemed futile or inappropriate does not abate with dissemination of further information or discussion.

Since the early 1960s, mostly in the United States and other Western nations, patient autonomy has been a major driving force—maybe even *the* major driving force—in all discussions about decision making in health care.[3] Although most people would not question the crucial role that patient autonomy plays in acceptance or rejection of treatment options offered, there is far less agreement regarding the role (if any) that respect for patient autonomy should play when the requested treatment is deemed medically futile.[4] At the heart of this debate lies the issue of what determines futility and who gets to define it.

Some authors have put forward the notion that the traditional physician's definition of medical futility completely disregards the notion that a medical treatment may in fact be useful in ways other than in terms of the strictly medical benefit it may or may not have for the patient involved.[5] As a corollary of such view, some have stated that patients are indeed entitled to care that is deemed by health care providers to be medically useless or only marginally beneficial.[6-8]

A large part of justifying this approach is the concept (stated or implied) that requesting futile treatment is not intrinsically harmful, and thus at worst it is a "morally neutral" proposition—that is, neither inherently unethical nor illegal. This is an extremely naive view of the problem. Many ICU therapeutic interventions are potentially dangerous and/or associated with the possibility of significant discomfort or even pain. Furthermore, in a world where health resources are unquestionably limited and finite, inefficient use of such resources is inherently and directly harmful, even when not to the patient, for such use is certainly harmful to all other members of society. Knowingly and voluntarily engaging in a potentially harmful activity with limited or no direct benefit to the patient is hardly a defensible position, even if the primary intention is not to cause harm.

Certainly all patients (and their families) are entitled to compassionate and respectful care—care that includes any and all interventions needed for enhanced patient comfort and in which measures to provide emotional support and help with coping issues are given the highest priority. However, there is no factual evidence or theoretical rationale to support the notion that agreeing to futile medical therapy is the only, or even the best, way for such emotional help to be provided. Thus, even if "futile" therapy may offer benefits other than those related to purely medical efficacy, these benefits could (and should) be achieved through other more appropriate means. That having been said, one must also acknowledge that in busy modern medical facilities where humanistic nontechnological (and thus nonbillable) aspects of health care are often totally neglected or given only a token importance, agreeing to inappropriate therapeutic interventions is often the most expedient way to resolve futility conflicts.

None of the physicians commenting on this case feel morally compelled to provide futile treatment to Patient B—even in an environment with infinite resources and no restrictions of any kind. What could be the rationale for such a decision? None of the 11 physicians elaborate on this, but one might speculate that there is the unspoken concern that the family's requests in such cases often reflect not the patient's best interests but the family members' own emotional and psychological needs and preferences.[2]

It is quite possible that in this utopia of unlimited resources, some physicians might react differently if the request were to come directly from a fully competent, rational patient. However, when dealing with a mentally incompetent patient who has no chance of recovering to competent cognitive life, physicians often find it impossible to believe that the individual would have freely chosen to be kept alive at all costs in such a dehumanized and irreversible state. In the presence of such deep-seated doubts, one finds it morally abhorrent to acquiesce to requests that are not in the patient's best interest or reflective of the true patient's preference.

For example, the parents who cannot cope with the idea of withdrawing the ventilator from their dying, comatose daughter riddled with metastatic cancer are acting out their pain, their sense of loss, and their denial of the inevitable, but they are hardly acting exclusively (or even mainly) with their daughter's well-being as the only consideration in the decision-making process. This is, of course, completely understandable and part of being human. However, as much as physicians sympathize with their plight and empathize with their pain and suffering, it is not ethically justifiable to engage in actions judged, to the best of the physicians' ability, to be of no possible benefit to the individual affected and that may in fact be harmful, dangerous, uncomfortable, or even undignified.

Patient B's case is one in which aggressive intensive care can be considered futile with virtual certainty. Absolute and complete certainty is neither achievable in real life nor a reasonable requirement for decision making. The old scientific ideal of *episteme,* or absolute certainty and demonstrable knowledge, is a lofty but unobtainable goal. As the philosopher Karl Popper[9] pointed out more than 30 years ago, "the demand for scientific objectivity makes it inevitable that every scientific statement must remain tentative forever." Thus, the word *futility,* in this medical context, does not refer to acts that are clearly impossible (e.g., decapitating a patient with a brain tumor and keeping him alive) or totally implausible at that particular point in time (e.g., transplanting all organs simultaneously in a patient with multiple organ failure). Rather, use of the term simply reflects an effort to achieve a result that, even if theoretically possible, available data and experience suggest is highly improbable.

For example, jumping without a parachute from a plane with a fire on board can be considered a futile effort to save one's life, despite the two or three reports of individuals whose parachutes failed to open but who still survived. Wanzer et al[10] stated that a rare report of a patient with a similar condition who survived is not, in and of itself, an overriding reason to continue aggressive treatment that is otherwise considered futile. Of course, the devil is in the details. What level of improbability defines futility? Less than 5%, less than 1%, less than 1 in 1000? What about cases in which the actual probability figures cannot be reasonably estimated because of lack of accurate data or at least sufficiently large prior experience? In addition, factors such as the complexity, risk, and cost of the contemplated intervention would also influence the likelihood that a therapy could be tried even if the probability of success is below the chosen threshold of futility.

Despite the efforts of many authors to determine what level of improbability equals futility, it appears obvious that this is a question with no single exact and correct answer. The medical profession can only propose a definition of futility, and ultimately society at large (or at least the local health community) will have to decide on the final operational definition.[5,11]

Finally, when making the decision regarding what constitutes appropriate care for Patient B, one must always keep in mind that a treatment that has a measurable effect on one part of the body is not necessarily "effective" or not futile. For example, take the case of a patient with anuric renal failure and an extensive hemorrhagic stroke. The family has decided against any form of dialysis. The patient has a small area of soft tissue infection, and treatment with antibiotics would be expected to eradicate this infection. Nonetheless, in the larger context of this case, such treatment can (and should) be considered to be futile therapy. Thus, the fact that physicians probably could, at least temporarily, improve some particular aspect of Patient B's deranged physiology is largely irrelevant to the overall determination that aggressive therapeutic efforts in this case are futile and therefore totally unjustified.

References

[1]Do-Not-Resuscitate Orders and Medical Futility. National Center for Ethics, Veterans Health Administration, 2000.

[2]Civetta JM: Futile care or caregiver frustration? A practical approach. Crit Care Med 1996;24:346–51.

[3]Schneiderman LJ, Jecker NS, Jonsen AR: Medical futility: its meaning and ethical implications. Ann Intern Med 1990;112:949–54.

[4]Jecker NS, Schneiderman LJ: Futility and rationing. Am J Med 1992;92:189–96.

[5]Loewy EH, Carlson RA: Futility and its wider implications: a concept in need of further examination. Arch Intern Med 1993;153:429–31.

[6]Perkins HS: Ethics and the end of life: practical principles for making resuscitation decisions. J Gen Intern Med 1986;1:170–6.

[7]Ruark JE, Raffin TA: Initiating and withdrawing life support: principles and practice in adult medicine. Stanford University Medical Center Committee on Ethics. N Engl J Med · 1988;318:25–30.

[8]Veatch RM: Justice and the economics of terminal illness. Hastings Cent Rep 1988;18:34–40.

[9]Popper K: The Logic of Scientific Discovery. New York, NY: Harper & Row, 1968.

[10]Wanzer SH, Adelstein SJ, Cranford RE, et al: The physician's responsibility toward hopelessly ill patients. N Engl J Med 1984;310:955–9.

[11]Schneiderman LJ, Jecker N: Futility in practice. Arch Intern Med 1993;153:437–41.

Should Patient B
Receive Critical Care?

Jean-Louis Vincent, MD

I believe that whenever a difficult ethical decision arises, as happens all too often in intensive care medicine, it is important to return to the four fundamental ethical principles: autonomy, beneficence, nonmaleficence, and distributive justice. Interestingly, the United Kingdom's Department of Health[1] guidelines for intensive care unit (ICU) admission specifically employ the ethical principle of beneficence: no patient should be admitted to the ICU unless he or she "can benefit from the care offered." Dr. Batchelor from the United Kingdom clearly believes such a condition is not met in Patient B's case.

However, although such principles appear clear-cut on paper, in clinical practice the borders are often blurred. Physicians' interpretations of the word *benefit* may vary; importantly, no one interpretation is necessarily right or wrong. Medicine attracts doctors of all ages, backgrounds, religions, and creeds, and these factors, combined with other facets including local policies, training, and the influence of national and international peers, will determine how an individual responds to a particular situation.[2] Even in the case of Patient B, for whom treatment is seen by most practitioners as futile, there are individual variations and emphases in the responses given, reflecting the different innate and developed characteristics and beliefs of the respondents.

For example, the doctors from Hong Kong, the Netherlands, and New Zealand all bluntly state that the patient should not and would not be admitted to their ICUs, whereas Dr. Kapadia from India is ready to provide "standard" ICU support with mechanical ventilation, vasoactive drugs, and so on. Dr. Roy-Shapira from Israel discusses at some length the religious and political reasons why he would go against his own gut feeling to disconnect the patient from the ventilator and instead continue limited care.

Interestingly, although *limited resources* is a term that attracts keen political and media interest, and attempts to "rationalize resource allocation" occupy increasing amounts of the ICU manager's time, in this case, resource availability made little difference in the way in which most doctors would have reacted; only Dr. Karakozov from Russia, faced with the possibility of being able to use for once in his life the most expensive drugs and equipment, admits that this would prove too much of a temptation and he would throw caution to the wind and make every attempt to save Patient B, regardless of the apparent futility of the situation. Intensive care resources are indeed limited, but with careful thought and restriction of those resources to patients who can indeed benefit, available funding can be stretched to its maximum capacity. It is well recognized that intensive care is effective,[3,4] but it is only so when applied to patients who will benefit; when resources are limited, offering intensive care to a patient for whom treatment is futile is a waste of funding that could be better used elsewhere or for a more deserving patient. Indeed, Dr. Streat from New Zealand expresses his belief that resources should never be so great as to allow society to expect ICU admission for this type of patient.

In his response to this scenario, Dr. Fisher from Australia briefly raises the specter of limited availability of beds. The importance of this issue varies according to the country, or even according to the particular area or hospital. In Europe, for example, 46% of doctors report that admissions are often limited by bed shortages, the figure being particularly high in the United Kingdom and countries of southern Europe (i.e., Greece, Italy, and Portugal).[2] The problem of limited availability of beds is likely to get worse as the number of ICU beds fails to increase in line with the increasing numbers of critically ill patients. This problem highlights the need for appropriate and enforced admission criteria, so that patients for whom treatment is futile are not admitted.

The ethical principle of distributive justice demands the fair allocation of resources regardless of age, wealth, creed, and personal position or prestige. It is interesting that the doctors from Russia and India both suggest that if the patient or his relatives were particularly wealthy or well connected, the patient would receive different treatment from that given to the "ordinary" individual. This influence of power is stronger in some cultures and for some individuals, but it is a very real issue. During a recent visit by a key world leader to a European country, a whole ICU and ICU team were reserved in case there was an accident or incident. Is this really distributive justice?

But how can one "diagnose" futility? Who is to say when administering therapy to a patient becomes a futile act? A therapy may have an effect, even a positive effect on some localized parameter, but if the treatment fails to improve patient status as a whole, it can be said to be futile.[5] In essence, then, intensive care provided to a patient who will not benefit from it can be said to be futile, although this certainly does not mean that such a patient may not benefit from other types of hospital or community care (e.g., palliative care). This patient is certainly not excluded from the four ethical principles; the rights of autonomy, beneficence, non-maleficence, and distributive justice all apply. Indeed, by not admitting such a patient, physicians are complying exactly with these codes. The rights and needs of the patient can be more adequately met elsewhere.

All the authors apparently agree in principle that Patient B does not merit intensive care, and yet none identify any objective measures on which their decision is based. Although Dr. van der Spoel from the Netherlands alludes to the Acute Physiology and Chronic Health Evaluation II score, it can be assumed that this is only to illustrate the severity of the disease state, not to advocate its use in the actual decision-making process. Indeed, no severity score should by itself be the grounds for denying ICU admission. Some patients with very severe physiological abnormalities (and thus by this measure with very limited chances of survival) may and should be admitted to the ICU (e.g., after severe polytrauma or for profound shock).

One of the problems with the word *futility* is that it has a bad press and is seen as a negative label; terms often used in association with a determination that treatment will be futile—*worthless, pointless, no purpose, no hope*—give rise to feelings of failure and to the inevitable (yet often unacknowledged) power and presence of death. The need to save life is ingrained in doctors from the earliest days in medical school. Little thought or time is given to teaching physicians how to prepare their patients, or their patients' relatives, for death.[6] To admit that a patient is dying somehow reflects one's failure as a physician, and the death of a patient can be associated with often completely irrational feelings of guilt and blame.[7]

In cases like that of Patient B, in which relatives demand that everything be done despite the obvious poor state of the patient, communication is all important, as indicated by several of the contributors. Adequate communication involves providing a clear, concise, and understandable summary of the situation; it does not necessarily mean consultation or discussion. Indeed, Dr. Burrows from South Africa states that a diagnosis of impending death is, in fact, a medical decision. Dr. Roy-Shapira from Israel goes so far as to say that when medical care is not indicated, as in Patient B's case, this is a medical decision and "neither the wishes of the patient nor those of his relatives are relevant"; in his ICU, there would be no consultation with the family, but there would be a full explanation of the decision and the reasons behind it. Emanuel and Emanuel[8] noted that patient proxies often have an inaccurate idea about what treatment a patient may wish for himself or herself.

There may be many reasons for this, including feelings of guilt about their relationship with the patient, fear of losing a partner or parent, and unrealistic hopes and aims. Thus, an important part of effective communication when relatives' and doctors' views are apparently in opposition is raising the possibility that perhaps what the patient really would have wished may not be what the relatives want, while acknowledging that their concerns and requests are understood and making clear that they are in no way being walked over by what is often claimed to be a paternalistic profession. Cultural differences also influence the way in which a family reacts to an illness, and communication with the patient and his or her relatives must take such issues into consideration.[9] By exploring the "everything must be done" request further, frequently one discovers that what the relatives really mean is that their loved one must suffer no pain and die comfortably. In cases in which a deadlock seems to have been reached between relatives and staff, an ethics consultation may be beneficial. Schneiderman et al[10] recently reported that such consultations resulted in shortened ICU stays and fewer life-sustaining treatments in the case of patients who ultimately died, and that these consultations were viewed favorably by those involved. However, none of the doctors weighing in on Patient B's case suggest their use.

The four key ethical principles go hand in hand and cannot be considered in isolation. For example, autonomy alone cannot drive the decision-making process; a patient may indeed request that everything be done, but if, as in this case, that patient is dying, then autonomy may be a possibility only if the other ethical principles of nonmaleficence are not followed. Dr. van der Spoel from the Netherlands extends this principle to the child, relating the story of a premature newborn who had many congenital defects and for whom an operation was denied against the parents' wishes. To operate would have been to comply with patient autonomy (in this case, the parents' request that the operation be performed). However, operating would not have resulted in beneficence, and it would have resulted in maleficence (because the infant would have undergone needless suffering) and in unjustified allocation of limited resources (ultimately, the infant would have died anyway).

This case demonstrates the importance of and justification for acting according to conscience, even if doing so is not in keeping with the family's wishes. In particular, as in Patient B's case, a physician may decide that a patient is beyond any reasonable hope but the family may persist in their request that everything be done. In extreme cases, when the relatives cannot be persuaded, patient transfer to another institution may be considered, to avoid further confrontation in a situation already fraught with emotion. Persisting with a particular course of action when communication and trust have broken down benefits no one; transferring or even being willing to transfer a patient to another team or unit can be sufficient to restore the relatives' faith in the medical profession and enable the process of communication to restart. A patient of ours with severe heart failure, a cerebrovascular accident with aphasia, and renal failure requiring extracorporeal renal support could not be weaned from mechanical ventilation because of her poor neurological status. The relatives requested transfer, hoping that in some way this would help their loved one. We discussed the limitations of intensive care for this patient, but the family insisted and she was transferred to a smaller, private, religious institution. She was surely going to die, but the family was happy that all had been done and their wishes had been respected.

I would like to briefly mention fear of litigation as a push in the decision-making process. Although not discussed in detail by the respondents, fear of legal action is mentioned in passing by several of the doctors. In Europe, medical litigation has not yet reached the levels seen in the United States, but Europeans are slowly becoming more litigation conscious. Defensive medicine, defined as the "ordering of treatments, tests, and procedures for the purpose of protecting the doctor from criticism rather than diagnosing or treating the patient,"[11] is not necessarily good medicine. Treating Patient B to avoid a potential lawsuit would only prolong suffering.

In summary, Patient B is almost universally seen to be nondeserving of intensive care. Individual differences and cultural influences affect the reasoning behind this decision and the level of care the doctors would or would not offer.

References

[1] Department of Health, NHS Executive: Guidelines on Admission to and Discharge From Intensive Care and High Dependency Units. London, England: Department of Health, 1996.

[2] Vincent JL: Forgoing life support in western European intensive care units: the results of an ethical questionnaire. Crit Care Med 1999;27:1626–33.

[3] Manthous CA, Amoateng-Adjepong Y, al-Kharrat T, et al: Effects of a medical intensivist on patient care in a community teaching hospital. Mayo Clin Proc 1997;72:391–9.

[4] Metcalfe MA, Sloggett A, McPherson K: Mortality among appropriately referred patients refused admission to intensive-care units. Lancet 1997;350:7–11.

[5] Schneiderman LJ, Jecker NS, Jonsen AR: Medical futility: its meaning and ethical implications. Ann Intern Med 1990;112:949–54.

[6] Simpson M, Buckman R, Stewart M, et al: Doctor-patient communication: the Toronto

consensus statement. BMJ 1991;303:1385–7.

[7]Buckman R: Breaking bad news: why is it still so difficult? Br Med J (Clin Res Ed) 1984;288:1597–9.

[8]Emanuel EJ, Emanuel LL: Proxy decision making for incompetent patients. An ethical and empirical analysis. JAMA 1992;267:2067–71.

[9]Vincent JL: Communication in the ICU. Intensive Care Med 1997;23:1093–8.

[10]Schneiderman LJ, Gilmer T, Teetzel HD: Impact of ethics consultations in the intensive care setting: a randomized, controlled trial. Crit Care Med 2000;28:3920–4.

[11]McQuade JS: The medical malpractice crisis—reflections on the alleged causes and proposed cures: discussion paper. J R Soc Med 1991;84:408–11.

The Yin and Yang of Critical Care
Utilitarianism Meets the Law of Supply and Demand

Ivor S. Douglas, MD

The mission of critical care has been likened to the eternal quest for balance: balance between the doable and the achievable; equipoise between the unquenchable desire to preserve the dignity, sanctity, and uniqueness of life (both physical and metaphysical) and the immutable, undeniable, and inescapable certainty of a patient's mortality. The 88-year-old Patient B epitomizes in a tangible and recognizable fashion the potentially weighty responsibility deferred to critical care providers—that of deciding whether to admit or to decline admission; to treat with the intention to cure or treat with the intention to comfort; and to respect individual and balanced patient-provider autonomy or exercise professional, often paternalistic, privilege by declining to treat or provide critical care.

I will review the intensive care specialists' responses to this challenging scenario, in light of prevailing health care economics and societal mores in each country. I will focus on the determinants of decision-making practices and differences of approach to the relationship of doctor, patient, and family (and by extension, societal accountability). This case illustrates the conflicting and charged relationship between the law of diminishing returns, on the systems level, and a humanistic therapeutic imperative, on the individual level. One may reflect on this problem using a dialectical approach[1]—that is, a reconciliation or synthesis of the scientific and artful balance required for humane, responsible, and outcomes-directed care. This strategy is essential for optimal critical care in technologically advanced health care environments.

I will argue that interpolating the rationale of this dialectic approach into an ethical decision-making framework is fundamental to the practice of critical care—regardless of the intensive care environment, health care system, or prevailing political or religious milieu. This strategy might be dubbed applied utilitarianism[2]—a recognition that an unfettered desire to provide the greatest good for the greatest number leads, inevitably, to circumstances of confusion and suboptimal outcomes for the critically ill patient. The responses of the various critical care physicians to the patient scenarios presented in this volume are defined by how much emphasis is placed by society on individual autonomy versus group benefit. When patients have access to critical care resources that by any measure are extremely unlikely to achieve the expected care goals, the entire premise of intensive care is undermined and the tenuous argument for the specialty's existence is gravely threatened.

In all 11 health care environments represented by the intensivists who responded to this scenario, aging populations, increasingly expensive diagnostic and therapeutic options, and a shift to preventive, community-based care are defining the prevailing health care settings. For some of these practitioners, notably those in North America, these realities have daily implications for care decisions. For others, particularly those in developing countries in Asia and Africa, the overwhelming press of poverty and the health care challenges of deprivation, emerging infectious diseases, and traumatic injury create a vaguely surreal and difficult-to-reconcile "freedom" in critical care decision-making. There is a glaring and contradicting irony between caring for terminally ill elderly patients using physiologically futile therapeutic interventions, in developed societies, and providing any level of critical care in developing countries. In countries such as South Africa and in parts of Asia, where there is an absolute dearth of suitable preventive and health-promoting services, the ethical challenges clearly extend beyond reconciling controversies in critical care: a pervasive lack of minimal housing, sewerage, and access to clean drinking water outweighs the philosophical debate being discussed here.

In reflecting on the specific responses of the individual clinicians to the plight of Patient B, one should not overlook these complexities. The balanced and ethically supported responses are clearly a synthesized reflection of each region's political, religious, and economic realities. Despite this, these clinicians share substantially similar visions of ethical decision making in circumstances of nonlimited resources and when decision making rests solely with the intensive care physician. Despite the variances in the definition of futility, this realization provides a reassuring and reasonable reference point from which to derive common principles for beneficent and responsible critical care. Truog et al[3] tellingly remarked: "Arguments based on the futility concept conceal many statistical and value-laden assumptions, whereas strategies based on resource allocation force these assumptions to be stated explicitly."

One of the least contrived, yet sophisticated, insights into the prevailing social mores and health care priorities of a society might be gained from medical students and recently graduated doctors. Young postgraduate physicians for the most part retain some motivational idealism, tempered by an acute sense of the extremes of critical illness and wary respect for the therapeutic limitations of intensive care. Their training exposes them to a broad range of clinicians, who frequently embody both the highest and lowest competencies in ethical and clinically rational evidence-based decision making. It is through this diverse clinical exposure that junior physicians refine their decision-making styles and their approaches to providing ethical health care.

In North America, Europe, and Australasia, junior physicians are frequently the immediate decision makers in the provision of intensive care for patients such as this 88-year-old man. They find themselves in the unenviable position of reconciling irresolvable and frequently conflicting pressures—from patients' families and caregivers (often to continue hopeless treatment) on the one hand, and on the other, hospital administrators and senior clinicians demanding shortened lengths of stay, accelerated discharges, and more tightly regulated accountability for prescribing and clinical care. The comments of the responding critical care physicians should thus be cautiously considered, given their frequently distanced position from the pithy realities confronting junior clinicians.

I presented the scenario of Patient B to resident house physicians and senior medical students rounding in the medical intensive care unit (ICU) at a large academic medical center in New York City. The case was presented immediately after a review of the care plan for a 93-year-old nursing home resident with severe Alzheimer's disease and emphysema who was intubated and was receiving mechanical ventilation for severe pneumonia and intractable septic shock. The patient lacked durable medical power of attorney or a designated health care proxy. Despite the recognition of physiological futility and a predicted mortality of more than 80% for the ICU admission, there had been no question of the patient's inalienable right of access to maximal critical care, including broad-spectrum antimicrobials, vasopressor agents, and an endorsement of full code.

The responses of the resident physicians to the management dilemma presented by Patient B were entirely consistent with their decision-making process for the patient they had just admitted. There was also the conflicting sense of practice versus pragmatism. These physicians expressed little doubt that they would give the patient 48 hours of maximal support before "capping pressors" and discussing do-not-resuscitate decisions with the next of kin—even in settings with nonlimited resources.

New York State is burdened by complex legislation that specifically prohibits withdrawal of mechanical ventilation from dying patients who lack a health care proxy and do not meet a "clear and convincing evidence"[4] standard of advanced intent to avoid prolonged mechanical ventilation. Withholding or withdrawing life support is therefore further complicated in the highly litigious New York health care environment. It is remarkable that initiating ventilatory support and providing access to intensive care would be limited by physicians practicing in the United Kingdom and former Commonwealth countries of Australia, New Zealand, and Hong Kong. There is a diametrically contrasting practice in the United States, the Netherlands, and India. In those countries, health system management is in the hands of private corporations and regional bodies. Physicians from those countries concur that Patient B would receive ventilatory support and critical care. The ultimate responsibility for limiting or withdrawing care apparently rests to a greater degree with the patient's family.

Across most cultures, it is broadly accepted that there is no substantial legal difference between withholding and withdrawing therapy. However, implementation of therapeutic withdrawal is fraught with perceived ethical difficulties, both for clinicians and families. As noted by Vincent,[5] physicians with a firm adherence to a religious doctrine, particularly those from southern Europe, are significantly more reluctant to consider withdrawal as an option for care of a dying, critically ill patient. To a great extent, it is this disconnection between the ethical-legal framework for withdrawal of care and the realities of implementation that led investigators in the Study to Understand Prognoses and Preferences for Outcomes and Risks of Treatments (SUPPORT) to conclude that there were major deficits in clinicians' understandings, expectations, and experiences of the dying experiences of their patients.[6]

It remains a matter of conjecture that the prevailing centralized health economy and management in these former colonial countries contribute significantly to the strategies those physicians use to justify their resolution of the dialectical tension in favor of aggressive resource restriction. Physicians who practice in nationalized or centralized health care environments frequently deride their North American and Asian colleagues. It is their contention that the accommodations that are made by these "soft" intensivists—to respect individual and family autonomy at the expense of achieving therapeutic end points—are unfounded expediencies that significantly undermine the measurable benefit of intensive care. The diagnosis-related group system of compensation has resulted in tracheostomy's being one of the most highly remunerated activities (ranging from $94,386 to $217,427) in the American system of medical care.[7]

Locally dominant spiritual adherences and practices have a significant impact on the patient and his or her family and on clinician perspectives and decision making. Whereas utilitarian existentialism seems to be the preponderant view of most of the responding physicians, it is by no means the prevailing worldview of their patients. The emphatic statement by the Israeli clinician, Dr. Roy-Shapira, that he would ideally withdraw care and institute palliative support with maximal sedation is entirely consistent with prevalent views in much of Europe. However, the resolution of the dialectical tension is complicated by a prevailing Jewish halakhic imperative not to withdraw a medical intervention once it has been initiated. This physician's somewhat cynical and expedient compromise is to support patients through periods of clinical "suspended animation," during which the goals of care are neither explicitly treatment for cure nor treatment for comfort. This challenging, though factual, scenario is incongruous with the long-term viability of critical care as a credible subspecialty. It has been suggested that providing accountable, dependable, and uniform care for extremely ill and incapacitated patients requires a boldness of commitment to rationalism. Reconciling this with (in Dr. Roy-Shapira's words) "local politics, peer pressure, and hospital policy" in order not to be fired is not a unique conflict for many who aspire to an abstract purism.

A further remarkable difference between several of the physicians commenting on Patient B's case lies in their approach to the relationship of physician, patient, and family—in particular, the extent to which patient and family wishes are considered as part of the decision-making process for end-of-life care. As noted by Cook,[8] the emphasis on a parental (formerly paternal) model (initially described by Emanuel and Emanuel)[9] places a weighty responsibility on the physician as guardian and advocate for the incapacitated patient. The physicians from the Netherlands, New Zealand, and Hong Kong indicate that this patient would never have been admitted to an ICU—suggesting an aggressive, engaging, and parentalistic approach. By contrast, the scenario of Patient B's case was sufficiently familiar to those physicians from the United States, Israel, the United Kingdom, India, and Russia to elicit remarkably different responses. These ranged from the extreme of "trust me, the all-knowing doctor," to negotiated withdrawal of care with "intuitively reasonable" family members, to negotiations with a surrogate health care consumer, with relatives armed with information about all the options and encouraged to make "rational" choices.

Clearly, these are all attempts to reconcile the eternal dialectic of critical care. Interventions chosen for the purpose of meeting humane, achievable goals for patients, families, and physicians are part of thoughtful critical care. Strategies that leave patients in the therapeutic limbo of goal-less life support seriously endanger the mission and enterprise of intensive care as a viable health care provision.

References

[1]GW Hegel: The Phenomenology of Mind. Translated by Baillie JB. New York, NY: Harper & Row, 1967.

[2]Mill JS, Bentham J: Utilitarianism and Other Essays. Edited by Ryan A. New York, NY: Viking, 1987.

[3]Truog RD, Brett AS, Frader J: The problem with futility. N Engl J Med 1992;326:1560-4.

[4]In re O'Connor, 72 NY 2d 517, 531 NE 2d 607, 534 NYS 2d 886 (1988).

[5]Vincent JL: Forgoing life support in western European intensive care units: the results of an ethical questionnaire. Crit Care Med 1999;27:1626-33.

[6]A controlled trial to improve care for seriously ill hospitalized patients. The Study to Understand Prognoses and Preferences for Outcomes and Risks of Treatments (SUPPORT). The SUPPORT Principal Investigators. JAMA 1995;274:1591-8.

[7]Data from Solucient. Available at: http://www.solucient.com. Accessed November 9, 2001.

[8]Cook D: Patient autonomy versus parentalism. Crit Care Med 2001;29:N24-5.

[9]Emanuel EJ, Emanuel LL: Proxy decision making for incompetent patients. An ethical and empirical analysis. JAMA 1992;267:2067-71.

Patient C

Treatment of a "Classic" Intensive Care Unit Patient

Mitchell Levy, MD

The Case

Many of the 11 intensivists contributing to this book comment on the inconsistencies in this patient report, and it is difficult to believe all the facts in this case. In particular, Patient C's various underlying disease states and abnormal laboratory values seem incompatible with a normal, alert mental status. His serum sodium concentration alone would lead a clinician to question his competency. The problem is not merely one of semantics. It raises the question of whether something has been missed. More importantly, it demonstrates the extraordinary difficulty one faces when trying to describe a patient for whom treatment is truly medically futile. In Patient C's case, in countries where futility is not physician defined, a clinician would most certainly look for surrogate decision makers to help with decisions regarding level of care. Does the patient have any family or friends who might be able to shed some light on his previously expressed wishes for care, given the possibility that he is not now competent for decision making?

Laying the Ground

To establish the context in which to view this challenging case, certain givens must be accepted[1-6]: 1) The health care system is facing financial challenges of historic proportions. 2) Patients and their families often are underinformed for the end-of-life decisions they face. 3) Many patients and their relatives have unrealistic expectations of aggressive interventions in the face of irreversible, critical illness. 4) Some patients and their families, even when fully informed, will demand care that caregivers deem medically futile. 5) Many physicians, when faced with a conflict between their assessment that aggressive care for a critically ill patient will be futile and the strong wishes of a patient to receive this aggressive care, will allow for a brief trial of aggressive intervention.

Futility

Certainly, Patient C's case raises the fundamental questions of how medical futility is defined and who has the authority to define it. I will address the philosophical underpinnings of futility later. There are other issues that should be addressed even before beginning to define medical futility. One important point to remember is that one must be careful not to use the exception to prove the rule. This case does not represent even a small minority of the cases seen in most critical care settings. Although demands for care deemed futile by caregivers are in fact made, they are rarely this extreme or unreasonable. Intensivists certainly face situations in which the patient's family is unable to accept the finality of a diagnosis, has unrealistic expectations about the likely benefits of aggressive care, and asks that care be continued beyond the point where most of the critical care team would stop. However, even these cases are not the majority. It is far more common that sensitive, careful, compassionate end-of-life conversations bring the family around to the consensus view of the team.[7]

I do not mean to suggest an idyllic view of futility, where everything works out and reason prevails. This is far from the truth. However, the case described is also far from the truth, and cases such as these should not be used to build policy and create laws. Patient C may certainly have demanded care that most physicians would consider futile or at least unreasonable. It is also true that the ability of societies, both economically developing and developed, to pay for unlimited amounts of expensive intensive care therapies is limited at best. The responsibility of intensivists is to act in the patient's best interest and, as much as possible, in accordance with the patient's expressed desire for care. However, as the conditions of patients change, so do the types of therapy that can be offered. Dialysis does not have to be offered to an unstable, dying patient, when there is no chance for survival.[8] In the current case, almost all the 11 contributors, regardless of their cultures' definitions of futility, agree that if this patient continues to deteriorate, which certainly seems likely, no further therapy can be offered and care will be withdrawn.

Futility and Education

The issue here is the relationship between individual rights and the needs of society. This is an age-old question and usually leads to endless debate and rhetoric. In many developing nations, in an environment of scarce resources, it becomes clear that offering care deemed futile by a consensus of caregivers is unacceptable. The challenges, which one then faces, are twofold:

First, how is futility defined? I will not attempt to define futility here;

it is discussed at length elsewhere in the book. It is exceedingly difficult to define relative medical futility, because this is based on the preferences and beliefs of individuals. As the contributors make clear, in many countries this definition is in fact left to the individual physician or the physician community. In other countries, however, the definition and the resultant decision-making are not left to physicians but instead are culturally or religiously determined.[9]

It seems logical and reasonable that these definitions be physician based. Unfortunately, physicians (at least in America) have not always represented themselves well as thought leaders and moral reference points. Greed, ego, elitism, and the pace of medical practice have led to insensitive and uncompassionate physician behavior. This has eroded public confidence in the trust between physicians and patients.[10-13] Can physicians be trusted to make the right decisions for families' loved ones? In some countries, this question is answered much differently today than 40 years ago.

The second challenge is education. The demand for care deemed futile by caregivers may be due to lack of education, not only of patients and their families but of clinicians as well. What is the root of the unreasonable expectations held by some patients and their families about the efficacy of aggressive interventions in the intensive care unit (ICU)? Could it be possible that patients and their families ask for futile medical care not only because they do not understand the limits of medical technology but because clinicians have failed in some way to develop a therapeutic relationship based on trust? Good end-of-life skills remain hard to find. Physicians receive little if any formal training in how to communicate, listen, and be sensitive to the needs of dying patients and their families.[14-16] Doctors often assume that simply caring about their patients guarantees that they will offer true, compassionate end-of-life care. In fact, this is not at all the case. As survey after survey demonstrates, patients and their relatives are unhappy with the care received in ICUs during the process of dying.[17] Inadequate communication with physicians and poor pain and symptom control are frequently reported by families whose loved ones die in the ICU.[18,19] Doctors cannot talk about responsibility to society and utilization of scarce resources without reminding themselves of the central role played by end-of-life skills. As physicians improve these skills, the public discussion about who makes the decision might be easier to manage. Intensivists know from their everyday interactions in the ICU that as trust is restored to the physician-patient-family relationship, these issues and many others become much more workable.

Education is important not only for the caregiver but for the public as well. Physicians often are confronted with families who make decisions and demand therapies on the basis of inadequate or incorrect information. Understanding the limits of treatment and complexity of disease is difficult for most patients under the best of circumstances, let alone in the midst of a crisis of grief and loss.[20,21] To shift the decision-making process and definition of futility into the hands of caregivers, thorough and widespread public education is essential. Intensivists know how much easier this difficult process becomes if they take the time to speak with families and bring them into a fuller understanding of the issues being faced by their loved ones. This often requires more time than ICU physicians feel they can spare, but it is an essential aspect to limiting care in a compassionate and effective manner.[22] Educating the public about the limitations of care can only facilitate this process.[23] Needless to say, there will still be patients and families who demand unreasonable care. One has to question whether this will become the minority of cases rather than the rule.

Consensus Among Contributors

There is often discussion about the vast difference between cultures in the approach to futility and intensive care. Yet several of the 11 contributors suggest remarkably similar approaches: a brief trial of critical care, most likely involving ventilation and administration of vasopressors, and then, if the patient deteriorates and is unable to participate in decision making, the physicians involved in his care become the decision makers (there being no family). This means that if it becomes clear that continued therapy has little chance of success, care is withdrawn.

Most contributors state that they would provide the same treatment in a limited and unlimited resource environment. That is, the decision to admit Patient C to the ICU and apply aggressive therapies would be based on the likelihood of success rather than the availability of resources. None of the contributors list any specific scoring system that they use or would use to determine relative medical futility. Most of them simply indicate that in their opinion, the patient has little if any chance of survival even with aggressive intervention.

Several of the intensivists acknowledge that if pushed—either by the patient's family or by primary consultants—they would provide some limited form of therapeutic trial. This would be done with the understanding that if the patient continued to deteriorate, care would be discontinued after a short period.

According to contributors from the United Kingdom, New Zealand, and the Netherlands—countries where decision making and the definition of medical futility rest with physicians—aggressive interventions would not be offered to this patient. Instead, several intensivists suggest that end-of-life conversations would take place with the patient and he would be transferred to a low-tech environment where he would receive supportive, compassionate care. These contributors indicate that a different level of care, rather than no care, would be offered to the patient. The clear identification of end-of-life care as an important therapy to be offered may be a result of the added responsibility that is taken on by physicians when given the role of decision maker.

Even in countries where medical futility and decision making are physician based, the final authority may be unclear. Several contributors mention that although they believe that this patient meets their criteria for medical futility, they would admit the patient to the ICU and use aggressive interventions if pressured by the patient's primary physician. In every instance, the contributors describe a time-limited trial of intensive care, followed by withdrawal of life support if unsuccessful.

Most of the contributors discuss the challenge of balancing physician-determined medical futility with compassion. At first glance, the case may seem quite straightforward, leading to withholding or withdrawal of aggressive, life-sustaining therapies and the provision of good end-of-life care. However, many of the ICU physicians indicate a clear and ready willingness to rethink the case in more optimistic terms, even accepting the possibility that the patient might recover. For all contributors, it is a question not so much of available resources and wasted finances as of doing the right thing for the patient. Dr. Roy-Shapira from Israel writes, "Broadly speaking, I would like to give this patient the benefit of the doubt. I am not sure that treatment would be futile, and I would need more time. I would admit the patient to the unit." This is the surprising twist: faced with a patient for whom treatment at first appears to be completely futile, many of the intensivists indicate a willingness to give the patient the benefit of the doubt and apply a brief trial of aggressive therapy.

The Challenge of High-Tech Critical Care

The responses of these physicians illustrate the fundamental challenge in this era of high-tech, expensive medicine. Many technologies reach the marketplace before adequate results from validation studies become available. Yet physicians—and, for that matter, the public—define good-quality care in terms of (at least in part) the technology of a given ICU or institution. This blind rush toward new technologies drives the cost of health care in general, and critical care in particular, to astronomical levels.[24] As

the cost of providing medicine becomes not only exorbitant but also pro-
hibitive for many hospitals and cultures, medical care becomes a luxury
rather than a necessity. This reality then directly conflicts with the natural
compassion that most physicians exhibit when confronted with extreme
disease and suffering. Can physicians afford their compassionate instincts?
If they cannot afford to extend aggressive life-sustaining care in the same
way as in the past, how is the decision to limit care made? Does the medical
community first simply acknowledge that it is not possible to pay for all this
health care, and then begin to ration according to the public will or the will
of physicians? What prognostic data can physicians use to inform the
decision to limit care? As these contributors demonstrate, doctors will often
choose to do more, not less, and give patients the benefit of the doubt, even
in countries where physicians are not paid more for doing more.

        Then how to proceed? Should the public be asked to decide what
should be offered, and when, and to whom? How will the public be led to
make an informed decision that could be translated into legislation? Clearly
these questions are not easily answered. More to the point, it must be determined whether there is indeed a problem. As mentioned earlier, perhaps this
is more a question of education of caregivers and the public. That is, should
a program be developed so that ICU physicians are thoroughly trained in
end-of-life skills that will engender trust and thus make life-limiting
decisions easier for patients and their families?[25] Rather than talking about
rationing and limiting access to care, should physicians instead be talking
about improving communication skills and engaging in conflict resolution in
difficult family situations?

        With regard to conflicts over levels of care offered to patients for
whom treatment is deemed medically futile by caregivers, it may be that a
significant proportion of such conflicts could be resolved through better
communication between physicians and patients and their families, leading
to a "community standard" of trust in the relationship with caregivers.

Conclusion

The remarkable aspect of the contributors' comments on this case is the
consensus and similarity. Even with widely different cultural norms and
community standards, some striking similarities emerge. Many of the
physicians indicate that a short trial of critical care therapy, when demanded
by a patient, a family, or another caregiver, might not be automatically
dismissed. Most of the contributors state that when they deem treatment
medically futile, they attempt to dissuade the patient from requesting aggressive care and they strongly suggest end-of-life care. Some contributors, in

cultures in which medical futility is physician determined, would offer supportive care only, regardless of the wishes of the patient. Both views represent the attitude of combining clinical experience with compassion in order to offer the appropriate care to the patient for whom treatment is medically futile. In some cultures, the decision clearly lies in the hands of physicians; in other cultures, decision making is patient directed. Yet the process does not appear to be so dissimilar in the majority of cases, such as the one presented here.

Several contributors make very strong statements about the intensivist being in charge and then make it clear that there is room for discussion with primary consultants, which might lead to admission and aggressive care. Is this the point at which the approach across cultures becomes very similar? Do not intensivists try to first convince patients and their families that further care is futile and will only prolong suffering and the inevitable? When confronted with a patient, family member, or physician who appears to make unreasonable demands, do not intensivists then try to educate and nurture the individual into rethinking his or her demands? But do not ICU physicians often give in, out of a sense of compassion and wishing to do the right thing, and admit these patients, for a limited period, and provide care initially deemed futile? Do not intensivists always balance compassion with futility and thus often provide care, however briefly, that they do not truly believe has a strong chance of success? The question becomes, how do clinicians balance their medical sense of prognosis, the wishes of patients and their family members, compassion, appropriate utilization of expensive resources, and appropriate utilization of scarce resources?

It may be that physicians oversimplify and undervalue the profound nature of this dilemma by viewing this as a matter of wasting valuable resources. The issue is so much more than an issue of money. How can physicians expect caregivers to be the only ones who define futility and make end-of-life decisions? The preferences of patients must be considered in a more formal way than leaving it up to the assessment of "good, caring physicians." Should the public be asked to decide what should be given, when it should be given, and who should receive it? How will the public be guided to make an informed decision that could result in legislation? If it is difficult for physicians to agree on the definition of medical futility, how can the public be expected to take on this difficult task? This dilemma seems to speak loudly to the need for a true partnership in the decision-making process—not by legislating the process into the hands of either the patient or the physician but by building, through trust, education, and perhaps legislation, a true collaborative process of end-of-life decision making.

References

[1]A controlled trial to improve care for seriously ill hospitalized patients. The Study to Understand Prognoses and Preferences for Outcomes and Risks of Treatments (SUPPORT). The SUPPORT Principal Investigators. JAMA 1995;274:1591–8.

[2]Prendergast TJ, Luce JM: Increasing incidence of withholding and withdrawal of life support from the critically ill. Am J Respir Crit Care Med 1997;155:15–20.

[3]Hickey M: What are the needs of families of critically ill patients? A review of the literature since 1976. Heart Lung 1990;19:401–15.

[4]Johnson D, Wilson M, Cavanaugh B, et al: Measuring the ability to meet family needs in an intensive care unit. Crit Care Med 1998;26:266–71.

[5]Singer PA, Martin DK, Kelner M: Quality end-of-life care: patients' perspectives. JAMA 1999;281:163–8.

[6]Faber-Langendoen K: A multi-institutional study of care given to patients dying in hospitals. Ethical practices and implications. Arch Intern Med 1996;156:2130–6.

[7]Nelson JE: Saving lives and saving deaths. Ann Intern Med 1999;130:776–7.

[8]Luce JM: Making decisions about the forgoing of life-sustaining therapy. Am J Respir Crit Care Med 1997;156:1715–8.

[9]Vincent JL: Forgoing life support in western European intensive care units: the results of an ethical questionnaire. Crit Care Med 1999;27:1626–33.

[10]Asch DA, Hansen-Flaschen J, Lanken PN: Decisions to limit or continue life-sustaining treatment by critical care physicians in the United States: conflicts between physicians' practices and patients' wishes. Am J Respir Crit Care Med 1995;151:288–92.

[11]Goold SD, Williams G, Arnold RM: Conflicts regarding decisions to limit treatment: a differential diagnosis. JAMA 2000;283:909–14.

[12]Lynn J, Teno J, Phillips S, et al: Perceptions by family members of the dying experience of older and seriously ill patients. Ann Intern Med 1997;126:97–106.

[13]Tulsky JA, Chesney MA, Lo B: See one, do one, teach one? House staff experience discussing do-not-resuscitate orders. Arch Intern Med 1996;156:1285–9.

[14]Solomon MZ: How physicians talk about futility: making words mean too many things. J Law Med Ethics 1993;21:231–7.

[15]Tulsky JA, Chesney MA, Lo B: How do medical residents discuss resuscitation with patients? J Gen Intern Med 1995;10:436–42.

[16]Danis M, Mutran E, Garrett JM: A prospective study of the impact of patient preferences on life-sustaining treatment and hospital cost. Crit Care Med 1996;24:1811–7.

[17]Jamerson PA, Scheibmeir M, Bott MJ, et al: The experiences of families with a relative in the intensive care unit. Heart Lung 1996;25:467–74.

[18]Hanson LC, Danis M, Garrett J: What is wrong with end-of-life care? Opinions of bereaved family members. J Am Geriatr Soc 1997;45:1339–44.

[19]Schechter NL: The undertreatment of pain in children: an overview. Pediatr Clin North Am 1989;36:781–94.

[20]Danis M, Federman D, Fins JJ, et al: Incorporating palliative care into critical care education: principles, challenges, and opportunities. Crit Care Med 1999;27:2005–13.

[21]Curtis JR, Patrick DL, Caldwell E, et al: Why don't patients with AIDS and their clinicians talk about end-of-life care? Barriers to communication for patients with AIDS and their primary care clinicians. Arch Intern Med 2000;161:1690–6.

[22]Tulsky JA, Fischer GS, Rose MR, et al: Opening the black box: how do physicians communicate about advance directives? Ann Intern Med 1998;129:441–9.

[23]Weeks JC, Cook EF, O'Day SJ, et al: Relationship between cancer patients' predictions of

prognosis and their treatment preferences. JAMA 1998;279:1709–14.

[24]Curtis JR, Rubenfeld GR (eds): Managing Death in the ICU: The Transition From Cure to Comfort. New York, NY: Oxford University Press, 2000.

[25]Brody H, Campbell ML, Faber-Langendoen K, et al: Withdrawing intensive life-sustaining treatment: recommendations for compassionate clinical management. N Engl J Med 1997; 336:652–7.

Should This Patient Be Admitted to a Critical Care Unit?

David Crippen, MD

The success of intensive care is not to be measured only by the statistics of survival, as though each death were a medical failure. . . . It is to be measured by the quality of lives preserved or restored, and by the quality of the dying of those in whose interests it is to die, and by the quality of the human relationships in each death.
—G.R. Dunstan, "Hard Questions in Intensive Care"

Patient C is a moribund patient with multiple system organ failure. He is in a clear death spiral but desires the application of life-support systems, despite the expressed opinion of critical care physicians that such care will do nothing but increase his discomfort during an inevitable dying process. With regard to the opinions of the multinational group of critical care providers, there seems to be a fairly clear division of labor along the lines of resource availability as well as of avoiding ineffective treatment. Physicians practicing in resource-challenged locales do not much buy into the concept of giving moribund patients the benefit of the doubt. Their threshold for accepting patients for resource-intensive care is fueled by the amount of resources that must be removed from others in the pool requiring them. They have been more or less empowered by their health care underwriters to prioritize admissions in terms of potential benefit, not necessarily patient desire.[1] Conversely, physicians in resource-rich countries buy heavily into the concept of individual patient autonomy,[2] the "right" to more or less unlimited medical care on demand.

For example, in India, where demand greatly exceeds supply, there are too many people and not enough assets.[3] Like most developed nations, India has a free, state-supported service, which necessitates being very resourceful because expending resources on one patient may affect others. And in such a system, there is both great benefit and great detriment. To a large degree, rationing occurs in a chillingly efficient and practical scheme. Those who cannot afford care feel the effects of rationing, but those who can afford it get world-class care. It is very much the survival of the fittest. Such a system forces prospective patients to plan very effectively for their care. It is necessary to set limits at the micromanagement level—the level of the consumer rather than of the provision system. Admitting nursing home patients with dementia in the terminal stages to an intensive care unit (ICU) simply does not happen, because that luxury cannot be afforded. Limits are placed on the duration of intensive care, and if there is not clear evidence of progressive benefit, such care is withdrawn quickly, so that the patient's family does not lose precious resources or go flat broke. Family conferences are held daily and include discussions about how cash reserves are holding up.

Similarly, in the United Kingdom, aggressive prioritization is necessary for resources to be available to the widest population. Daniels[4] looked at the difference in allocation of scarce resources in the United Kingdom and the United States. Annually, the British spend less than half what Americans spend on medical care, but the former provide universal access to the system for all citizens, and all know in advance what limitations are in effect. Advanced planning not only is possible—it is mandatory. Because all patients have equal access within this closed system, resources must be allocated with judgment regarding which resources are most beneficial for the entire group. Introduction of beneficial new procedures must be weighed against the benefits of alternatives. Although an added service or procedure might help one group of patients, its cost might be high enough to deny other patients services. Because the best care is provided by distributing the resources most equitably within the system, saying yes instead of no might be unjust. Physicians do not directly or indirectly benefit from delivering care at lower cost; thus the incentive to provide it is limited.

Conversely, medical care in the United States is an open system.[5] No prospective medical budget determinations or estimates of cost-effectiveness are made. All varieties of medical care are equally funded in theory, but there is a catch-22. Instead of determining how much should be allotted to services, the United States health care system prospectively allows all services and then denies reimbursement for some after they have been rendered. This unusual tack has several implications. One is that caregivers are placed in the position of expending resources that may not be replenished, on the whims of gatekeepers and because of technicalities. Another implication is that there is no real way to determine whether resources expended will be replenished until after the fact, which makes prospective planning difficult if not impossible. Accordingly, resource allocation in the United States proceeds according to a table of organization that is poorly responsive to need and very sensitive to demand.[6]

America is predictably the only country in the spectrum of those represented here that routinely accepts these patients for ICU treatment.[7] The reasons are multiple. There is an incentive to treat anyone for anything as long as a bill can be sent to a third party that has an obligation to constituents it knows little or nothing about. Also, patients in the United States believe they own the health care system and can demand and obtain as many services as they want for as long as they want, with no proof of need.[8] The questions that then need to be explored are, how does this socialization affect the ability to provide adequate care to a large population, who pays for it, how long can the health care system afford to do it, and, of course, does such a policy really improve the health of Americans compared with how other countries do it with more prioritization policies?

It is a common complaint of critical care providers that resources are "wasted" on patients in the ICU for whom treatment is deemed futile— patients that are predicted to do poorly in the face of continued aggressive care. A substantial amount of literature supports the premise that such care is expensive out of proportion to benefit. Scheffler et al[9] found a nonlinear, U-shaped relationship between use of resources and probability of survival. At one end of the spectrum, an increasing amount of therapeutic intervention generated a decreasing mortality rate. At the other end, 40% of resources were used to prolong life temporarily in 9% of the patient population, and the mortality increased as the number of therapeutic interventions increased. Detsky et al[10] found that patients having the highest hospital expenses, on average, fell into two groups: survivors who had been predicted on admission to have a poor chance of survival and nonsurvivors who had been predicted on admission to have a good chance of survival. Patients having the lowest charges were found to be nonsurvivors who were predicted on admission not to survive and survivors who were predicted on admission to survive.

There does not seem to be much difficulty identifying which patient population can be predicted to benefit from the allocation of scarce resources.[11] The problem is how to efficiently divert resources from patients who are predicted to do poorly and toward those who are predicted to do well. A crucial issue to explore is the benefit, if any, of giving lots of scarce and expensive health care to Patient C. Is this the right thing for a society to do in an age of increasing population and decreasing resources? Does Patient C deserve to have as much spent on him as he desires—or does he have an obligation to die in order to make way for use of resources to benefit many patients who are more needy?

Traditionally, the culture of physicians has been to do everything possible for the patient and damn the resource utilization. In the old days, physicians protected their patients from fear of the unknown where the only thing they really could offer was unflagging moral support. That support was intensified by unrelenting advocacy for patient wishes. Recently, physicians have been seeing themselves as protecting patients from the gatekeepers who would deny them their due, to save money for the stockholders.[12] But as technological advances allow physicians to maintain vital signs indefinitely, there develops an inevitable inconsistency in terms of what is clinically effective in prolonging sentient life and sustenance of vital signs in a warm cadaver.[13] On the one hand are the hopes and desires of medical consumers; on the other hand is the ability of physicians to sustain but not reverse organ system failure. The case of Patient C highlights this difference.

For the purposes of this discussion, I will take a different tack than that taken by previous discussants. I will paint a word picture of this patient as if he actually exists. I will present this patient as he would likely be dealt with in the average community-level tertiary referral center for medical-surgical patients presenting with acute illness in the United States. This patient is an amalgam of several patients I have dealt with as director of an ICU. The scenario that follows occurs every day in hospitals throughout the United States and most definitely in the hospitals I have been involved with. I have stylized a physician response to illustrate the reality of ICU resource allocation where patient autonomy supersedes clinical reality. Here is how this case might have progressed in real life:

Patient C said he wants everything done. I approached him at the bedside about the issue of his demands. I said, "I must truthfully tell you that there is no further treatment for your disease process. We have exhausted all possible recourse and you are in the terminal phase of AIDS [acquired immunodeficiency syndrome]. You were diagnosed with AIDS in 1989, you have survived longer than many, and now you have entered the terminal phase and there is no respite for your multiple organ system failure. The reality is that you will die very soon and nothing can stop it."

He replied, "I don't want to die and I want everything done." As far as he was concerned, it was up to him to decide whether to die on the ventilator with full life support, and if he wanted this care, it was his right to have it, with no justification needed, and it was my duty to provide it on request.

My clinical opinion was that intubation, mechanical ventilation, dialysis, and unlimited use of blood products and other ICU resources would not appreciably alter his death spiral. After due consideration, I refused to provide them to the patient, because they would make him more uncomfortable and not alter the death spiral. These things would interfere with my ability to provide comfort, which was my prime motivation in this case. I told him, "You knew this was coming. Why didn't you make arrangements for this time long before now? You could have chosen hospice as an effective comfort measure. That information was available to you. That you didn't choose that option in no way obligates me to provide hospice in an intensive care setting." The patient was then transferred to a ward bed while receiving a morphine infusion and died in fulminating multiple organ system failure an hour later.

A full range of players, including the hospital administration, nurses, and housestaff, were upset that a patient's desires were not fulfilled, and the case was referred to the hospital ethics committee for a retroactive ethics consultation. This meeting was deemed educational and not punitive and was open to all the administrators, nurses, and housestaff and to ethicists in training. Some interesting comments were made by those at the meeting.

The hospital administration considered this a customer satisfaction issue. All things being equal, the administrators believed that a satisfied customer was a business asset. Their position was that whatever it took to make the patient happy was good business. They were very concerned that a customer desired a hospital service and was denied that basic right. In their opinion, provider staff should always err on the side of the maxim "The customer is always right." An unhappy customer yields problems far worse than the problem of keeping him or her satisfied. That there was no benefit, and considerable potential discomfort, did not enter into it.

A third-year internal medicine resident got up and made the sweeping statement that any patient in this or any other institution had a right to any treatment he or she wanted, money was no object, and no physician had any authority to tell the patient otherwise. "It is my job to do whatever patients think will benefit them," she said. It is a basic right of living in a civilized society that can afford to spend billions of dollars a year on empty-calorie snack foods.

The floor nurses were upset that the patient did not go to the ICU. They thought that it was inappropriate to put the patient in an "isolated" area of the hospital, because the nurses "couldn't take care of him adequately there." He wanted everything done and they could not do "everything" where he landed. They equated comfort care with doing nothing. He wanted something done and so they needed to be doing something, and what they thought they needed to be doing could be accomplished only in an ICU, where his care could be closely monitored. Their perception of the ICU was as a place that both uses high technology to reverse organ system failure and provides high-tech hospice on demand. They believed, in essence, that the ICU is a place to do more while doing less, because if the staff is not doing everything, it is being remiss in its obligation. Using the general medical floor as a hospice and instituting a morphine infusion titrated to comfort is not enough.

Then came the social activists seeking out discrimination against socially disconnected patients. One went so far as to say that my description of the patient's living conditions before admission showed I was judgmental. Never mind that it was part of a full history and showed the patient's expectations for the end of his disease process. Was it not true that I actively discriminated against this patient because I considered him a social pariah with an unfashionable sexual preference and a negative value–laden disease? What if this exact scenario had involved a well-connected captain of industry with a full family? Would I not have fallen all over myself to do anything he wanted? Never mind that all patients in this category need planning for hospice long before the terminal event.

There was in fact no evidence of sexual or social discrimination in Patient C's case. We have admitted patients with alcoholic cirrhosis and active gastrointestinal bleeding to the ICU on numerous occasions and considered their fate using the same criteria as those used for Patient C. I had invoked the concept of medical futility in diverting this dying patient from an acute care area. When the hospital ethicist, an academic with a PhD in medical ethics, asked if I could have prolonged the patient's life a finite period by intubating him and putting him on dialysis, I had to answer in the affirmative. The ethicist was uncomfortable with this decision. He thought that the situation might not be adequately covered by the rubric of medical futility. If it was possible to keep the patient alive for a variable time by intubating him and putting him on dialysis (for his fulminating hepatorenal syndrome and coagulopathy), then such treatment technically was not futile and I might be obligated to give it on demand because it was the patient's right as an autonomous citizen. I could refuse to use life-supporting hardware only if doing so would not prolong his life at all.

At this point we got into a semantic squabble about exactly how long Patient C's life would have to be prolonged before treatment could be considered futile. The ethicist thought that prolongation of life for seconds or minutes, but not hours or days, indicated futile treatment, but I never pinned him down to an exact time to the second. The patient wanted to live a little longer on machines, and it did not matter what his reasoning was. It was my duty and obligation to give it to him. But there were other clinical problems involved in prolonging his life on machines. It would have been necessary to restrain and sedate him to facilitate using this hardware, and to painfully poke holes into him for catheters. After institution of such treatment, it would have been necessary to act in a very aggressive manner to decrease not only the discomfort of his terminal disease process but also the additional discomfort I conferred on him by machines that only prolonged the inevitable. I tried to put it in better perspective for the ethicist by stating it differently: "The addition of life-supporting hardware capable of temporarily sustaining vital signs would not under any circumstances alter the death spiral. It would alter only the physical habitus of the patient as that spiral progressed."

The ethicist seemed a little more comfortable with that and wrote an opinion that basically said there was no real negligence or fault in this complex situation. Here is the text of his opinion:

> There are two separate questions here. First, what were the wishes of Patient C and was he competent to understand what he wanted and why? Second, was further treatment medically futile? The chart gives no indication that Patient C was incapable of making decisions about his treatment. It does seem that on a number of occasions he said he wanted everything done. On the face of it, this would seem to suggest that his wishes ought to have been followed. Yet there is a greater degree of complexity here than is evident on the chart. It seems from the chart that he did explicitly ask the staff for (potential) CPR [cardiopulmonary resuscitation] and mechanical ventilation as his death spiral tightened. But the attending physician reports that when he initially explained that these treatments were simply not going to be helpful, the patient seemed less insistent on them for a while. This adds a degree of uncertainty with regard to exactly what he wanted. Clearly he wanted to be cured and to get better and he did not seem to understand that this was not a viable option. When a staff member asked him if he wanted everything done, he said yes. But this may have meant he wanted everything done that might make him better, or it may have meant he wanted everything done that would extend his life even for a short time, or he may even have meant he wanted everything done that medicine could do, regardless of the possible risks and benefits. It was not clear what "everything done" meant to Patient C or even that it meant the same to him over the hours of his presence in the hospital. So the question of what Patient C wanted and whether he was able to understand his condition and the risks and benefits of possible treatment options remains unclear.
>
> The chart is again confusing concerning the issue of medical

futility. Court cases and debate among ethicists and physicians have seemed to result in an agreement that medical futility cannot be based on low quality of life or low probability of success. If a treatment has a reasonable chance of prolonging life, then a patient may request it even if the physicians think it is inappropriate. Although not all agree with this conclusion, it has become the standard for now. Although hospitals could establish public policies that they do not use certain life-sustaining treatments for certain patients with certain prognoses (e.g., we do not ventilate persons with hepatorenal failure, or we do not feed patients in a persistent vegetative state), none to my knowledge have done so, doubtless because of the difficulty of getting agreement on which treatments in which cases are medically futile. Hence, as long as a treatment is likely to prolong a patient's life to some reasonably significant degree (no one has defined this, but it seems that a few days might be considered reasonably significant to some people, whereas a few hours would seem not to be, unless there was some event of importance that these hours would permit for the patient), the patient may demand it and the physician seems bound to offer it, or to transfer the patient to a physician who will honor the patient's wishes.

But there are cases of true medical futility. That is, there are treatments that are contrary to the standard of medical care. These should not be offered even if the patient requests them. Two criteria are usually proposed to determine whether a treatment is medically futile in this strict sense. First, if a treatment cannot accomplish physiologically what it is supposed to accomplish, it is futile and must not be given. Second, if a treatment is irrelevant to a dying patient's major condition—such that, though it might treat an irrelevant minor condition (for example, fix a tooth), it will not prolong life—then the treatment is futile and must not be given. Note that the phrase here is "must not." It is not "need not." Medically futile treatments are contrary to the standard of medical practice. They *must* be forgone. Doing them suggests perhaps that a doctor or a hospital is more interested in making money than in treating persons.

In the case at hand, the attending physician's explanation was that the requested treatments would have been medically futile in this strict sense. Patient C was imminently dying from hepatorenal failure. Dialysis is not an option in such cases. Transfer to the ICU, together with mechanical ventilation, would not have prolonged the patient's life even a short time, in the physician's medical judgment. On the basis of this judgment, the physician refused to order these procedures. Mechanical ventilation would have done nothing to reverse or to postpone the dying process caused by the hepatorenal failure. The Ethics Committee agrees that, assuming the medical judgments the physician made are correct, the treatment modalities he rejected were indeed futile.

In the end, the ethicist agreed that the treatment Patient C desired was, at least by a stretch, futile according to the classic definition, but I know he thought in his heart of hearts that the patient's desires should have been granted, on humanitarian grounds. It was physically possible to prop the patient up for a variable period longer. It should have been his right, living as he did in a society that spends huge amounts of money on other totally frivolous endeavors, including pet rocks and Cabbage Patch dolls. The relatively small amount of money spent to ensure that his autonomy was not compromised pales into insignificance when one considers the amount of money the populace cheerfully spends to view rich sports professionals perform. Medical futility is never an issue until the procedure in question will not prolong life at all (or for some unacceptably brief but undefined period). However, the ethicist and I agreed that my actions were very acceptably sheltered under the rubric of medically inappropriate treatment. It was clearly medically inappropriate to accede to his wishes, even if treatment was not medically futile.

But that is an issue that is very hard to defend in actual practice. If you ask the hospital administration what medically appropriate care is, they will tell you that anything is appropriate that brings patients in, separates them from their insurance companies' money, and makes them happy so they will come back. If you ask the nursing staff, they will tell you, "Whatever prolongs the patient's life as comfortably as possible." If you ask the house-staff, they will tell you, "Whatever gets the patient's desires met." If you ask health insurance executives, they will say whatever gets them out of the hospital as quickly as possible.

The ethicist decried current definitions of futility that mandate that caregivers maintain vital signs as a proxy for life, but he saw no practical way out of it until public (and legal) perceptions should change. He felt strongly that if there is a (vanishingly small) chance that a patient might improve (for a variable time) with a procedure or treatment that physicians predict will not be of value, the patient must be given the opportunity to make that choice. He then quickly added that the patient should also bear the responsibility for the cost thereof. This magnanimous gesture sounds great in ivory-tower academia but it has a lot of associated problems in real life. All people who make such requests expect their insurance companies to fund them, or expect the hospital to eat the cost. And their invariable response to anyone who suggests that they undertake financial responsibility for personal preferences is, naturally, "That's discrimination."

Patient C had hopes and desires at the family practice level of medicine. He wanted to step into roles as if in a theatrical play, in which reality did not enter into the script. He wanted someone to tell him something that would make him feel better, when in reality there was no such advice available. He wished to step out of his unfortunate reality into a more pleasing fantasy. But just outside that fantasy lies the reality that intensive care is uncomfortable and expensive. If there is no appreciable discomfort associated with the application of life support, what is the need for titrated analgesics and sedatives? If the patient's end is to be marked by the administration of analgesics and sedatives, what is the problem with administering them in a non–intensive care setting? Can he not be made as comfortable without the high-tech hardware? The end result will be the same. The ICU is ostensibly a place where a high-tech care plan is applied for the reversal of organ system failure. Is the ICU also a place to necessarily palliate the dying? Why do so in the ICU? Does the benefit justify the resource utilization?

I have intentionally painted a picture of us (ICU physicians) versus them (everyone else involved in intensive care) because the issue looms large in the field of intensive care. Accumulating experience suggests that the future is clear for the problem of prioritizing death spirals in acute care units. It comes down to a Mexican standoff about what constitutes appropriate care in your—the intensivist's—unit. There will be only one party in charge—them or you. There will not be any gray area. If it is you, then you will tell the patient what resources are available. If it is them, they will tell you what resources will be mobilized. It is like a negotiated settlement in wartime. The only property that is ever negotiated is the property no one cares anything about. If it is valuable property and someone wants it bad enough, the combatants will eventually start killing each other for it, and then winner takes all. You are willing to accede to some of the patient's demands because you feel sorry for him and you want him to feel as though you are fully supportive. That is the negotiated settlement. But there is a point in his demand schedule beyond which you are probably not willing to go. It is at that point when you find out who is in charge.

Patient C and others like him are either "appropriate" candidates for expensive and resource-rich critical care or not.[14] That judgment will be based either on their desires as autonomous citizens or on whether therapy that can benefit them requires the unique intensive care environment.[15] If you put a patient in an ICU simply because he or she desires it and a bed is available, no insurance reimburser in the world will pay a nickel for that decision. Is his vision of "everything possible being done" a primary goal in intensive care medicine? What if he told you he really, really wanted to ensure that no stone was left unturned in the search to find *anything* that might keep him alive a few more hours but regrettably he had no ability to replenish resources expended? Suppose he said he just would not feel right about the experience unless he died with the maximal application of everything possible. And what if he asked you to list *any* therapy that might accomplish that goal, and you said, "Well, we could put you on extracorporeal membrane oxygenation and it would prolong your life a bit." If his response was, "I want it. I'll feel better knowing that everything possible was done for me," would you arrange it? Probably not.

Futility is defined different ways by different people, depending on their motives. If a patient demands that I bore a hole in his head with a power drill to let out evil vapors, I do not have to do it, because it really is futile. Supposing a woman who had a lumpectomy and radiation therapy for breast cancer 5 years ago lands in your ICU with terminal metastatic disease everywhere. Bilateral lung snowballs. Then she says that not only does she want intensive care, she wants a bilateral mastectomy for completeness. Would you grant her the mastectomy just because she desires it? Probably not. However, if one of my patients with a progressively fatal disease demands to be intubated to prolong life, I do not have the authority to resist that request, because it is not futile by current definitions. Intubating him will indeed prolong his vital signs, the current definition of life, and is thus not futile treatment. If it prolongs his vital signs, it is effective treatment. Never mind that it will only prolong the dying process in a much more uncomfortable mode. Anything that is capable of prolonging vital signs is fair game until the definition of futility is altered.

There are several problems associated with dealing with medically inappropriate care in the ICU that require effective redress. Whether to intubate the patient just mentioned on demand is not really a viable clinical issue. I am currently mandated to intubate him on demand as long as doing so has the potential to keep him alive in some sense for a longer period than if I did not.[16] I am mandated to continue mechanical ventilation only until a second echelon of futility has been reached. When I have demonstrated that such treatment is ineffective in reversing the progressive disease process, I may then discontinue his mechanical ventilation and render comfort measures.[17] This is perhaps a subtle distinction, but it is an important one in a society in which individual autonomy talks and paternalism walks.

In fact, there was no need to "abandon" Patient C in the sense of parking him in a corner and ignoring him. The nuts and bolts of effective palliative care in the ICU are well represented in the literature.[18] What he needed he would not have received any better in an ICU than in a hospice, which is where he needed to go.[19] The big break point here is an interesting question. Does a frightened, uninformed, and unsupported dying patient in an irreversible death spiral necessarily feel better when his vital signs are prolonged at his request?[20] What is the time frame for when "critical care" becomes futile? Minutes, hours, or days? Clearly one cannot mount a "medical futility" argument on longevity in and of itself. There is some limit that everyone will agree to. However, I would not put a 90-year-old patient who had dementia in the terminal stages on extracorporeal membrane oxygenation after no response to 1 hour of CPR. That is medically futile. It is the gray area that demands further investigation. The number of families and patients who demand futile care because they are out-and-out manipulative or crazy is relatively small. It is that population that needs some encouragement, in the form of aggressive persuasion, to do the right thing. The majority of "futile" care is demanded by well-meaning patients and families who think that what they are doing is right because they get little or no guidance otherwise from their personal physicians.[21] Part of the job description of full-time, dedicated critical care physicians in charge of their ICUs is dealing with these issues with patients and families. When ICU directors are in charge, intensive care is rendered more effectively.[22] By extrapolation, end-of-life care can be handled more effectively as well. A lot of patients and families receive diffident and ineffectual advice, or no advice at all, from their doctors on end-of-life issues, prompting the patients and their relatives to take the path of least resistance. When ICU directors become in charge of ICUs, there is a strong potential to improve end-of-life care within the continuum of intensive care.

References

[1]Streat S, Judson JA: Cost containment: the Pacific. New Zealand. New Horiz 1994;2:392–403.

[2]Crippen D: The current state of critical care medicine. Cost Qual Q J 1998;4:5–7, 10.

[3]Singh M: Ethical considerations in pediatric intensive care unit: Indian perspective. Indian Pediatr 1996;33:271–8.

[4]Daniels N: Why saying no to patients in the United States is so hard. Cost containment, justice, and provider autonomy. N Engl J Med 1986;314:1380–3.

[5]Crippen D: Rationing and regionalisation of health care services: a critical care physician's opinion. Clin Intensive Care 1992;3:100–6.

[6]Crippen DW: Emergency medicine redux: the rise and fall of a community medical specialty. Ann Emerg Med 1984;13:539–42.

[7]Osborne M, Patterson J: Ethical allocation of ICU resources: a view from the USA. Intensive Care Med 1996;22:1010–4.

[8]Crippen DW: Emergency care or convenience care. Providers may have to choose one hat. Postgrad Med 1986;80:107–9.

[9]Scheffler RM, Knaus WA, Wagner DP, et al: Severity of illness and the relationship between intensive care and survival. Am J Public Health 1982;72:449–54.

[10]Detsky AS, Stricker SC, Mulley AG, et al: Prognosis, survival, and the expenditure of hospital resources for patients in an intensive-care unit. N Engl J Med 1981;305:667–72.

[11]Clermont G, Angus DC: Severity scoring systems in the modern intensive care unit. Ann Acad Med Singapore 1998;27:397–403.

[12]Curtis JR, Rubenfeld GD: Aggressive medical care at the end of life. Does capitated reimbursement encourage the right care for the wrong reason? JAMA 1997;278:1025–6.

[13]Crippen D, Whetstine L: ICU resource allocation: life in the fast lane. Crit Care 1999;3:R47–51.

[14]Zoloth-Dorfman L, Carney B: The AIDS patient and the last ICU bed: scarcity, medical futility, and ethics. QRB Qual Rev Bull 1991;17:175–81.

[15]Whetstine LM, Crippen D: Desire vs. need in the medical marketplace. Cost Qual 1999;5:31–3.

[16]Dugan DO: Praying for miracles: practical responses to requests for medically futile treatments in the ICU setting. HEC Forum 1995;7:228–42.

[17]Crippen D: Terminally weaning awake patients from life sustaining mechanical ventilation: the critical care physician's role in comfort measures during the dying process. Clin Intensive Care 1992;3:206–12.

[18]Crippen D: Practical aspects of life support withdrawal: a critical care physician's opinion. Clin Intensive Care 1991;2:260–5.

[19]Danis M, Federman D, Fins JJ, et al: Incorporating palliative care into critical care education: principles, challenges, and opportunities. Crit Care Med 1999;27:2005–13.

[20]Schneiderman LJ, Gilmer T, Teetzel HD: Impact of ethics consultations in the intensive care setting: a randomized, controlled trial. Crit Care Med 2000;28:3942–4.

[21]A controlled trial to improve care for seriously ill hospitalized patients. The Study to Understand Prognoses and Preferences for Outcomes and Risks of Treatments (SUPPORT). The SUPPORT Principal Investigators. JAMA 1995;274:1591–8.

[22]Field BE, Devich LE, Carlson RW: Impact of a comprehensive supportive care team on management of hopelessly ill patients with multiple organ failure. Chest 1989;96:353–6.

Multiple Organ Failure
and Intensive Care

Richard Burrows, MB, BCh

"All is flux" (Heraclitus). There is no fine line that differentiates one action from another. Disease may be mild, moderate, severe, intractable, or irreversible, with no precise distinction between the various grades. Dying too is a process with no precise moment that divides alive from dead or when the process is irreversible as opposed to reversible.

Improved technology in intensive care has meant that patients who some years ago would have been expected to die can now be treated and return to active lives. However, inabilities to define the moment of death have also often led to nothing more than protracted death on machines or "successful" resuscitation that is meaningless and leads to nothing more than a life of vegetation. As part of this uncertainty, terms such as *unreasonable, reasonable, ordinary,* and *extraordinary* become part of the jargon that everybody appears to understand but that defies precise definition. Uncertainties are an integral part of medicine and are what make decisions necessary if day-to-day management is to proceed.

There is a perception that the physician acts as a godlike, paternalistic figure, making no decision other than to engage in a constant struggle against the certainty of death, with scant regard to the fact of death as anything other than a failure. This attitude, it seems, must be curtailed, and this can only be achieved by the patient or his or her surrogate, who must place limits on the physician to avoid treatment the patient or surrogate considers unnecessary. Where the refusal to undergo certain forms of treatment is concerned, the issue is clear and the patient's refusal to undergo treatment is paramount and has consistently been supported by the courts. The issue is less clear when the patient or surrogate wishes to press for treatment. It seems obvious that when presented with the option of a lingering death, the reasonable patient or surrogate would prefer to avoid the option. This is true for the most part, but occasionally the opposite seems to be the case, as surrogates press for treatment with little or no chance of success. The reasons surrogates should object to the cessation of treatment are several, including the fact that physicians have difficulty communicating with them effectively as outlined in a report of the Study to Understand Prognoses and Preferences for Outcomes and Risks of Treatments (SUPPORT).[1] Such behavior on the physician's part (which may, in large part, be driven by an unreasonable fear of litigation) cannot be condoned, because it is destructive to any physician-patient relationship. Nonetheless, assuming relatives and patients have been fully informed, there are two concerns that run counter to the decision on the part of the patient to force treatment. When treatment is not expected to achieve any reasonable outcome (i.e., when treatment is futile), it must be refused; and when a lack of resources forces rationing, treatment must be refused as well.

A decision is a deliberate choice between options of varying probability, and it helps to understand how the individual arrives at a decision. Broadly, decisions are made on two levels. They are logically arrived at, on the one hand, and, on the other, are made by a subconscious method that appears to be intuitive but that in fact is dependent on past experience and training.[2] George Bernard Shaw[3] wrote: "There is a point at which the most energetic policeman or doctor, when called upon to deal with an apparently drowned person, gives up artificial respiration, although it is never possible to declare with certainty, at any point short of decomposition, that another five minutes of the exercise would not effect resuscitation." Under these circumstances, all medical personnel make the same decision at one time or another. Logical deduction will tell the physician that a few minutes of hypoxia will lead to irreversible brain damage and thus there is little point in continuing. When the point of decomposition is more distant, the uncertainty clearly becomes greater, but once again the physician's training, along with discussion with colleagues, will allow him or her to develop an opinion that further treatment will be of no benefit to the patient and the physician may well decide that it would be futile even to attempt cardiopulmonary resuscitation in the first place. This is no different from a firefighter who uses his or her acquired skill and decision-making ability to make decisions regarding how long to continue fighting a fire when lives either of fellow firefighters or of persons in the building have been lost.

The very severe shortage of resources—in particular, the shortage of intensive care facilities in South Africa—is illustrated by the following figures relating to the intensive care unit (ICU) of Addington Hospital in Durban. There were 525 admissions to this 8-bed ICU in 2000. However, 410 other patients were refused admission to the ICU in that same period. In 95 of these cases, admission was refused because the medical staff believed that intensive care would be futile. Seventeen patients could be managed on the general ward and did not require ICU admission. The bulk of the patients (298) were refused admission because the unit was full. Many of these patients were transferred at state expense to other institutions, including private ICUs, at clinicians' insistence that treatment continue.

The equivalent of US$6.7 million was spent on 100 consecutive patients in a surgical ICU. Forty percent of this was spent on patients who subsequently died. It is doubtful that any economy can stand this level of expenditure for any length of time. It is an impossible consideration in South Africa and is even worse in other African countries, where medical facilities hardly exist. There must be a rationing of sorts, which Pellegrino[4] defines as "diagnostic elegance and therapeutic parsimony."

Patient C is positive for the human immunodeficiency virus (HIV) and is clearly in the final stages of acquired immunodeficiency syndrome. In 1999, the World Health Organization[5] estimated that 33.6 million people worldwide had the disease. A total of 23.3 million of these people were in sub-Saharan Africa. The problem is overwhelming.

The level of services that should be brought to the populace is a complex issue that society at large has to address through administrators and politicians, with advice from those working with patients, but there is simply no possibility that all these patients can be treated in ICUs as part of their dying process. The physician can only decide whom to treat on the basis of the likelihood that the patient will survive the hospital admission. All that can be reasonably asked of the physician is that he or she approach each case fairly and without prejudice. Many patients with limited life spans are admitted to ICUs (e.g., patients who have undergone cancer surgery or patients with chronic airway disease). The only sane way to deal with such admissions is to prognosticate on the probability of surviving or not surviving hospital admission, and act accordingly. Although patients and their relatives should have information concerning resources and can be offered alternatives if they can afford them, and although it is best if they concur with decisions made, it is simply not possible to allow them to dictate all decisions concerning withdrawal of treatment.

The question of the level of service that must be delivered to the individual to save his or her life has been addressed in South Africa.[6] The renal program, like intensive care, is hopelessly oversubscribed. Medical criteria for allowing a patient to remain in the program in KwaZulu-Natal include the following: no significant disease elsewhere (e.g., cerebrovascular disease), no evidence of malignancy or previous noncompliance with medical treatment, adequate vision, negative HIV status, and normal liver histology if hepatitis B surface antigen positive. Patients older than 55 years are enrolled only under exceptional circumstances, if they are candidates for renal transplantation.

A patient who was undergoing chronic dialysis was found to no longer meet the criteria for continued chronic dialysis and was consequently removed from the program. He mounted a legal challenge to the decision:

> The applicant broadens his attack and contends that the State is constitutionally obliged to accommodate his emergency medical treatment and is constitutionally obliged to provide the means with which he can receive emergency medical treatment in accordance with the provisions of section 27(s) of the Bill of Rights contained in Chapter 2 of the Constitution of the Republic of South Africa, Act 105 of 1996. The applicant concludes with the following allegation:
>
> "I have been advised and verily believe that the State is not possessed of infinite resources where (sic) which to treat indigent citizens such as myself. I do however aver that the State, as author of the Constitution and the ultimate respondent herein, has an express constitution (sic) duty to render life-saving medical treatment to me. I challenge and attack any statement on behalf of the State that it is directing sufficient resources to the provision of emergency medical treatment."[6]

The court summed up further:

> In conclusion the applicant states that he is not asking that the state provide him with the best and most expensive medical treatment that science has been able to devise but is simply requesting any form of treatment which will have the effect of prolonging or saving his life.[6]

The court noted the severe lack of resources facing the medical services:

> The Clinic services the whole of the Province of KwaZulu-Natal and also patients from the Eastern Cape. Of all the patients who require haemodialysis, only 30% can currently be treated. The other 70% have been refused treatment.[6]

The court noted too that the department has to provide, within budget, health care from primary through tertiary and above and that it has to carry out a balancing act when allocating money for each service. Making funds available for the renal program would simply mean that funds would be denied elsewhere. If the department were forced to treat the patient, another patient who complied with the guidelines and had a better chance of survival because he or she qualified for transplantation would be denied treatment.

The South African constitution states: "No-one may be refused emergency medical treatment." It was argued that the patient would die very shortly if he did not receive the medical treatment and was therefore in the category of patients in need of emergency medical treatment. Thus the state, having created the right, must provide the funds to allow effect to be given to such right. But an emergency just like anything else is a matter of degree and cannot force the individual physician to act to save a patient's life unless there is an indication that the life can be saved.

In discussion, the court stated:

> The case made out by the applicant mirrors what at present seems to be a popular conception that the rights created in the Bill of Rights are absolute and can be exercised and enjoyed without limitation. This is of course not so. The rights are by section 36(1) limited in terms of law of general application to the extent that the limitation is reasonable and justifiable in an open and democratic society. The rights are also limited by the rights of others. A right extends only so far as the point to where it does not infringe upon another person's right.[6]

Similar sentiments were expressed in the English Court of Appeal:

> I said that there were two distinctions between the prohibition on violating the person and the duty to provide care and assistance. So far I have mentioned only one. The second is that while the prohibition on violation is absolute, the duty to provide care is restricted to what one can reasonably provide. No-one is under a moral duty to do more than he can or to assist one patient at the cost of neglecting another.[7]

Also, the court expressed the opinion that the decision to deny treatment was not a function of the court:

> Insofar as the present case is concerned, however, I am of the view that it is not the function of the Court to decide who shall and who shall not receive the required medical treatment. It is for the medical practitioners to make these decisions. They are qualified, whereas I am not, to decide on clinical grounds which patient will

benefit the most from the treatment. The Court will only interfere if
the doctors involved have exercised their judgement unreasonably,
arbitrarily or have discriminated against a patient.[7]

The decision not to offer dialysis to a patient when dialysis might give
the patient some remaining life is extraordinarily difficult, but it cannot be
simply ignored. It must also be recognized that there is a problem when the
physician allows himself or herself to be the servant of two masters—the
coffers of society and advocates for the patient.[8] Although the physician
must work within the system and must therefore be cognizant of the
shortfall in resources, it does not follow that he or she should be the
agreeable agent of the administration in applying rationing. The physician's
primary consideration should be what it has always been—the patient.
However, there cannot be absolute advocacy, especially when the physician
must choose which patient to treat because available resources do not extend
to the treatment of all. It serves no purpose to refuse to deal with the issue,
and all the patient should expect is a decision of fairness without prejudice.

Infection with HIV brings with it some special problems not obviously apparent where patient C is concerned. In South Africa, many patients
present with no clear indication of their HIV status, and it has been asked
whether testing positive for HIV should mean refusal of admission to the
ICU.[9] Confidentiality is regarded as vitally important, and the need to maintain confidentiality is strengthened by the principle that no patient should be
forced to be part of something that may disadvantage him or her. Many
other patients with equally fatal diseases are admitted to the ICU for
treatment, and to refuse admission solely because the patient tests positive
for HIV cannot be justified. Also, confidentiality is vital because of society's response to the disease. More sophisticated communities may be better
able to deal with people who are HIV positive or may simply be more
sophisticated in their persecution. In South Africa, however, a young woman
who admitted her status was stoned to death by a prejudiced mob. There is
therefore good reason for laying down strict rules concerning the approach
to patients who are HIV positive. Nonetheless, the problem of making reasonable decisions in the face of uncertainties still remains.

Patient C has entered the terminal phase of the disease and can be
expected to die shortly. No amount of technology thrown at him will alter
this fact. From a medical point of view, ventilation and other intensive care
measures are not justified. Comfort care is all that should be offered.

Basing legislation on such a case—legislation allowing the physician
to withdraw therapy despite objections by the patient's family—might be

said to be "bad law." But it seems that society's insistence that autonomy is always right in all circumstances has accomplished that objective anyway! Many relatives are little concerned with the fact that insistence on continued treatment may put other patients at disadvantage. But even if it is agreed that patients and families should maintain autonomy over their decisions, it cannot be allowed at the expense of the lives of others. Some type of legal balance appears necessary.

Where there is a consensus on forgoing treatment, the issue is clear when the patient is competent and aware. Treatment may not be forced on him or her, even if refusal of treatment means the patient's death. Information from surrogates may make the patient's wish to forgo treatment clear, although the existence of an advance directive does not guarantee clarity. The decision-making process is far less clear when the patient or surrogate presses for treatment judged by the medical attendants to be of no benefit. In this sense, the medical decision is not an ethical one—it is simply a decision based on the probability that the patient will die after admission.

Although it is reasonable to question the ethical nature of any decision to stop resuscitation, ethical analysis has been criticized as failing to solve the problem. There is a spectrum of consent, from uninformed to totally informed. Ethical principles can be only a guide, with no precise answer or direction, and ethicists have noted that precise ethical decisions are too much to expect from bioethics.[10] Placing excessive burdens on the principles of autonomy, beneficence, nonmalfeasance, and justice risks making these principles unsustainable—expected to solve problems rather than form a framework of understanding. Physicians are often accused of arrogance, and ethicists may have the same human failing. Ethicists may have an ax to grind and may spread a patina of impartial analysis over their support of a particular position, thus destroying any real progress. Certainly, physicians have interpreted patient values using their own values and education in ethics, and perhaps legislation has driven home the fallacy of such an attitude, but patients have consequently been forced to make medical decisions that they are simply not trained to make. Clinical problems can be as intractable as moral problems, and the clinical problem of when to stop treatment cannot be solved by application of a moral directive to the exclusion of clinical considerations that can be dealt with only by clinicians.

The decision to withdraw treatment is onerous and is affected by, among other things, the patient's wishes, surrogate requests, legal perceptions of what is permissible, and medical perceptions of what is practicable.

It serves little practical purpose to insist that physicians turn over this decision to the patient, his or her surrogate, or the courts. Like the South

African court, the (United States) President's Commission for the Study of Ethical Problems in Medicine and Biomedical and Behavioral Research[11] insisted that

> the question [of not resuscitating] is not one for judicial decision, but one for the attending physician, in keeping with the highest traditions of his profession. It is a question peculiarly within the competence of the medical profession of what measures are appropriate to ease the imminent passing of an irreversibly, terminally ill patient in the light of the patient's history and condition.

Likewise, the Vatican declared:

> For such a decision [the decision not to resuscitate] to be made, account will have to be taken of the reasonable wishes of the patient and the patient's family, and also of the advice of the doctors who are especially competent in the matter. The latter may in particular judge that the investment in instruments and personnel is disproportionate to the results foreseen. . . . They may also judge that the techniques applied impose on the patient strain or suffering out of proportion with the benefits which he or she may gain from such techniques.[12]

Having relatives make medical decisions to stop resuscitation is fraught with difficulties, and in fact, there is evidence that they do not want to make such decisions,[13] and asking them to do so merely puts the burden of responsibility (guilt?) on their shoulders. Their unwillingness may be due to a variety of reasons, including guilt, loss of trust in the medical staff, reluctance to accept the medical opinion that treatment is futile, and religious or cultural beliefs. These may result in an insistence that resuscitation continue to the exclusion of all other considerations. It appears that trust is most destroyed when the relatives believe that the physicians are not being honest with them—that is, the relatives think either that the physicians are protecting the relatives from themselves or that the physicians believe that the decision to stop resuscitation will have repercussions.

The notion that everything possible be done in the ICU is particularly difficult, given that mortality rates for many common problems in the ICU have remained constant despite the advent of new and expensive therapies, which themselves are questionable, with little support in the literature on evidence-based medicine.[14] Asking a patient's relatives to decide under these circumstances is asking them to make a decision that the physician should have already made, and consent under these circumstances is nothing other than an emollient of consciences of the medical staff.

The South African Law Commission,[15] in its discussion paper entitled "Euthanasia and the Artificial Preservation of Life," set out a possible mechanism for dealing with patients who are terminally ill:

> If the chief medical practitioner of a hospital, clinic or similar institution where a patient is being cared for is of the opinion that the patient is in a state of terminal illness as contemplated in this Act and is for this reason unable to make or communicate decisions concerning his or her medical treatment or its cessation, and his opinion is confirmed in writing by at least one other medical practitioner who has not treated the person concerned as a patient, but who has examined him and who is competent to submit a professional opinion regarding the patient's condition on account of his expertise regarding the illness of the patient concerned, the first-mentioned medical practitioner may, in the absence of any directive as contemplated in section 6(1) and (2) or a court order as contemplated in section 9, grant written authorisation for the cessation of all further life-sustaining medical treatment and the administering of palliative care only.

The document, if it is to be accepted, will have to be accepted in its present form, which includes provisions for active euthanasia. Because active euthanasia is currently unacceptable, the bill has remained stagnant. Thus, legal authority to make a medical decision to withdraw treatment is unlikely to be granted in the near future.

When the medical staff have been open and honest with them, most patients and families will usually accept the inevitability of the outcome and concur with the decision. However, this is by no means always the case, and there is a very real need to give some sort of legal authority to physicians to make the reasonable clinical decision to discontinue treatment in the ICU in the face of unreasonable, unwavering resistance by relatives. This would allow the reasonable clinician of integrity to provide the best care, within the confines of available resources, for all his or her patients. Those with incurable diseases would not be exposed to prolonged suffering, and other patients would be given the best chance for survival. It is a question of finding the reasonable balance between patient (surrogate) authority and physician authority, with due regard to the demands of society. The alternative is an ethical and legal fraud, in which medical staff must act in a furtive manner to deliver the service as reasonably and equitably as possible.

Do not try to live forever. You will not succeed.
—George Bernard Shaw, *The Doctor's Dilemma*

References

[1]A controlled trial to improve care for seriously ill hospitalized patients. The Study to Understand Prognoses and Preferences for Outcomes and Risks of Treatments (SUPPORT). The SUPPORT Principal Investigators. JAMA 1995;274:1591–8.
[2]Klein G: Sources of Power: How People Make Decisions. Cambridge, MA: MIT Press, 1999.
[3]George Bernard Shaw: The Doctor's Dilemma. Edited by Landes W-A. Studio City, CA: Players Press, 1997.
[4]Pellegrino ED: Rationing health care: the ethics of gatekeeping. J Contemp Health Law Policy 1986;2:23–45.
[5]WHO World Health Report. December 1, 1999. Fig 99000-E-1.
[6]*TS v Minister of Health:* Province of KwaZulu-Natal.
[7]Hoffmann LJ, in Airedale NHS Trust v Bland: a judgement of the Court of Appeal, reported in (1993) All ER 821 at 857 B.
[8]Levinsky NG: The doctor's master. N Engl J Med 1984;311:1573–5.
[9]Bhagwanjee S, Muckart DJ, Jeena PM, et al: Does HIV status influence the outcome of patients admitted to a surgical intensive care unit? A prospective double blind study. BMJ 1997;314:1077–84.
[10]Toon PD: After bioethics and towards virtue? J Med Ethics 1993;19:17–8.
[11]President's Commission for the Study of Ethical Problems in Medicine and Biomedical and Behavioral Research: Deciding to Forego Life-Sustaining Treatment: A Report on the Ethical, Medical and Legal Issues in Treatment Decisions. Washington, DC: U.S. Government Printing Office, 1983.
[12]Paris JJ, Reardon FE: Moral, ethical, and legal issues in the intensive care unit. J Intensive Care Med 1991;6:175–95.
[13]Shade SG, Muslin H: Do not resuscitate decisions: discussions with relatives. J Med Ethics 1989;15:186–90.
[14]McIntyre RC, Pulido EJ, Bensard DD, et al: Thirty years of clinical trials in acute respiratory distress syndrome. Crit Care Med 2000;28:3314–31.
[15]South African Law Commission: Euthanasia and the Artificial Preservation of Life (Discussion Paper No 71, Project No 86). Pretoria, South Africa: South African Law Commission, 1998.

General
Multidisciplinary Survey

Discussion of the
Medical Aspects of Futility

David Crippen, MD

It would be thought that a form of government based on individual rights and organised by reasonable people would result in a society less contentious than currently is the case. Reasonable people, it would be thought, would understand the need for individuals to tolerate each others needs and indeed to develop an understanding of the mechanisms wherein society can only function in an aura of tolerance. But the opposite appears to be the case. Pecuniary interest in consumer society has destroyed tolerance, setting individual against individual in a competition that inevitably must fail to look after the weakest in society.
—George Bernard Shaw, *The Doctor's Dilemma*

The clinical accuracy of peer-reviewed medical literature is evolving rapidly and with it the potential to learn a great deal about achieving benefit in critical care.[1] The advent of the Internet and electronic bulletin boards led to real-time contact with a multinational pool of working physicians, as well as up-to-the-minute data regarding patient care on a multinational platform.[2] This has created a new global medical village, in which the furthest citizens reside just around the corner. In 1994, CCM-L (http://ccm-l.med.edu), the first medical bulletin board dedicated to the specialty of critical care medicine, was founded. At the time of this writing, a multinational contingent of about 1000 CCM-L subscribers, including physicians, pharmacists, nurses, other interested providers, medical ethicists, and researchers, access a sophisticated mail server located at the University of Pittsburgh in Pennsylvania. About half live and work outside the United States. The purpose of CCM-L is to provide a forum to discuss, and to maintain a data bank for, the holistic daily care of the patient as it pertains to the intensive care setting. Included in the discussion are problems associated with limitation, withholding, and withdrawal of life support. CCM-L provided the platform from which the opinions that form this work were drawn.

Looking over the analysis of the treatment approaches described by the multinational panel of 11 critical care experts, I found some interesting trends. Global resource allocation for critically ill patients tends to proceed along the lines of what is available regionally to support it. Countries with few available resources tend to allow physicians in the trenches to micromanage resource allocation for the most expensive consumers. The populations in those countries are accustomed to prioritization of services. Availability of excess for entitled individuals on demand is a rarity. Conversely, individuals in more affluent countries consider access to expensive resources a basic societal right—a prerogative that is sometimes legally enforced. There is ample suggestion that critical care is expensive, but there is little if any evidence that affluent societies cannot afford it. They simply choose to allocate their resources according to political goals, some more effectively than others.

With regard to medical practice in the United States, there is no scarcity of opinions on the relationship between resource allocation and utilization. Hiatt[3] wrote: "As we develop more and more practices that may be beneficial to the individual, but not to the interests of society as a whole, we risk reaching a point where marginal gain to individuals threatens the welfare of the whole." In a 1984 congressional report, it was stated that "the best responders are patients with acute reversible illnesses without significant underlying disease. The worst responders are patients with exacerbations of chronic conditions for which there is no definitive therapy."[4]

Philosophers naturally wax philosophical. In his examination of resource allocation "rights" at the macro level, Engelhardt[5] used the word *lottery* to imply that resource utilization is a matter of luck, not predetermination. The term *social lottery* suggests that some citizens are rich and prosperous and some are poor and have no influence, and that these conditions are randomized according to luck, because a person cannot pronounce his or her social condition at birth. The term *natural lottery* suggests that some citizens enjoy good health and some do not, again a situation in which the affected individual has little influence. Winners of the natural lottery are healthy; losers get sick. Winners of the social lottery have resources to pay for their health care; losers do not. Accordingly, it is unfair if citizens are not granted their legitimate rights, conferred by society, to adequate health care. This unfairness should be rectified by formal societal programs financed by contributions from all. Other citizens' desires may not necessarily be guaranteed by society. It is unfortunate if a citizen living in a Bowery slum cannot be treated by a surgeon in an ivory-tower medical center, but it is not necessarily unfair. It is an "unfortunate" lack of access that implies bad luck and does not compel compensation, only charity.

Bureaucrats look at the problem from a political perspective. Their view is that bad health does not permit citizens to pursue life, liberty, and happiness as (seemingly) "guaranteed" by the Constitution. Lawmakers believe that if one could define health care as a basic right, the next step would be to make it a legal right, and then access would be mandatory for all. At least one legislator (Representative Jesse Jackson) has promoted a constitutional amendment decreeing health care a constitutional right.[6] The wording of the bill is ideological: "All citizens of the United States shall enjoy the right to health care of equal high quality and Congress shall have the power to implement this article by appropriate legislation." Unfortunately, this proposal provides no realistic plans for distribution of and payment for these services. If such idealistic resolutions were adopted, the same public that demands affordable health care indemnification would then have the right to as much care as they liked, but there would be no logistical way to obtain this care and no clear funding to support it. The potential for lawsuits would be endless, and each successful legal action would require providers to render care with dubious hope of reimbursement. So far, all of these requests have been rejected by the courts, and there are currently no legal rights to health care in the United States.

The issue of meaningful access to medical care is a problem. Everyone agrees that it would be a great thing, everyone desires it, but no one can decide what sorts of basic medical needs and demands should be indemnified and who should be eligible to receive them. If unlimited and first-come-first-served access—especially to expensive, highly technological care—is freely granted, the resulting demand crushes any resource pool. Some kind of prioritization scheme is necessary to match supply with need. Traditionally, the criteria used to identify and prioritize potential health care consumers have been based on some degree of utility.[7] It makes no sense to underwrite access to expensive and scarce resources if the patient will not benefit from it. Therefore, some kind of formal or informal prioritization is brought to bear that identifies, even roughly, those with a potential to benefit and necessarily excludes those that cannot. But it must be remembered that utility means different things to administrators of resources and persons desiring to obtain them. For a consumer of medical services, need for those services exactly equals his or her desire. Health care consumers do not like to be told that their particular complaints have been weighed in a balance and found wanting. The person who goes to an expensive emergency department with a trivial complaint says, "It's an emergency to me" (ergo someone else should underwrite the cost). If access is prioritized, no matter how creatively, someone somewhere will be excluded, and history has shown that this person will move to have his or her exclusion set aside by lobbying or legal maneuvers. As more potential consumers are excluded to conserve resources, the administrative costs to maintain their exclusion as they fight to get back on board the overcrowded boat increase commensurately.

It is difficult enough to get potential consumers to line up in some sort of order amenable to prioritization (trying to herd cats comes to mind), but the issue is further complicated by the availability of machines that support but do not necessarily reverse organ system failure, and by the difficulty in knowing how to apply them.[8] The medical literature suggests that it is hard to predict specifically who will benefit from expensive intensive care, especially in the initial stages of a disease process.[9] It is frequently necessary to give the benefit of the doubt to patients who are seemingly poor choices for treatment and to apply aggressive care until failure becomes obvious, lest a substantial number of apparently moribund patients who may respond to treatment be lost for lack of accurate outcome predictability. Severity-of-illness scoring systems accurately predict outcome only for rather large groups.[10] Large groups are collections of individuals, and so in the end, scoring systems can be relied on only as statistical models of how things might be if one lived in a perfect world. In a perfect world, no rational person would allow himself or herself or loved ones to endure life-in-death on mechanical life-support systems if there was no compelling hope of return to a healthy, functional state. And yet, seemingly rational people demand frequently that physicians do just that.[11] Why?

It is emotionally easier for a patient and a patient's family to make decisions about withholding care if they perceive an associated bad outcome.[12] When so informed, they are less likely to feel that they are "killing" the patient. If the perceived outcome is death (even if resuscitation should be performed), then it is not a big stretch to allow that inevitable death to happen earlier rather than later. However, once life-supporting care is instituted, a much more complex picture of potential outcome appears. The patient now has survival options he or she did not have before resuscitation took place. Once this occurs, more complex choices must be made. Patients and their families are forced to look at the reality that their decisions are inextricably linked to an outcome that is no longer inevitably fatal. They now control variables that may hasten death rather than avoid its prolongation. This is a subtle but exceptionally important point. Instead of yielding to inevitable death, life-support systems provide the potential to manipulate the logistics of death, and a large number of families find those options less difficult and less disturbing than letting go. That is why the issue of futility in high-tech medicine has been forced to the forefront.

Critical care physicians are prepared to use life-sustaining technology when the benefit seems to outweigh the risk and when there is a reasonable chance of an outcome that the patient would desire.[13] Decisions to place patients on life support are usually hastened by expectations embellished by the emergent nature of the proceedings. It frequently seems reasonable to buy time, using the most invasive life-support technology, to see if the disease will respond to aggressive treatment. If, however, organ system failure proceeds to irreversibility, the reasoning behind life-support technology becomes moot, and such technology serves no further useful function. Physicians must then be prepared to remove supportive technology when it appears, in their best judgment, that inevitable death rather than meaningful life is being prolonged.

But there is a problem with this seemingly logical rationale. The general public is aware that current technology is capable of indiscriminately maintaining some of the vital functions of the body, but critical care physicians know that the same supportive technology does not necessarily heal disease processes. An unintended side effect of modern technological advances has been the plausibility of maintaining moribund patients in a state of suspended animation for prolonged and sometimes indefinite periods.[14] Families of moribund patients perceive them as being stalled in comfortable suspended animation, awaiting the miracle of reanimation. Critical care physicians perceive them as not being alive, in the sense of enjoying life, and not being able to die, because technology has temporarily arrested the disease process but not the disease. In many cases, reanimation of such patients is impossible, even with the advanced medical technology available. Yet their families are content to await the elusive miracle.

The courts have repeatedly affirmed the authority of surrogates to regulate medical treatment, regardless of their reasoning.[15] When a patient becomes incapacitated, surrogates are granted virtually unlimited power to dictate treatment options if they claim proximate knowledge of what the patient would want, were he or she not incompetent. This position is based on the postulation that any attempt to interject physician paternalism into the equation of surrogate decision-making is ethically unacceptable. But even in the best of circumstances, families of moribund patients have difficulty making critical decisions regarding life-support systems, because of the complex information that must be assimilated and comprehended. Families frequently cannot understand the difference between allowing a patient to die from untreatable disease processes and hastening death by some therapeutic or antitherapeutic maneuver. Life-support technology can give the appearance of viability when in reality there is none once the machines are removed.

Under the current rules, surrogates do not have to proffer any reasoning or rationale, other than hope, for demanding futile life support. Some families believe that if life-support systems can maintain vital signs for a day or a week, suspended animation should be possible indefinitely. These opinions are frequently supported by articles in the popular press describing patients who awakened after years of coma. The only means used to determine utility is to ask, will this treatment result in sustained vital signs? Virtually any treatment that sustains vital signs is fair game, even if it will do nothing to revitalize the patient. The following line of reasoning— "We don't want a patient to actually die, because we find it emotionally disquieting; therefore, we are willing to alleviate our suffering by avoiding the moment of truth indefinitely"—is perfectly acceptable under the current health care system. There is a strong incentive to give the great lottery wheel a spin and try your luck. If you lose, you get nothing, but you do not lose anything either. If you win, your moribund relative gets a free intensive care nursing home. Surrogates have little incentive to authorize withdrawal as long as the patient does not look uncomfortable and there is the vanishingly small possibility of eventual success.

This situation seems to cry out for some kind of regulation to avoid excesses. There is evidence in the literature to suggest that futile care is dispensed (in some form) in the practice of clinical medicine, but no one knows how to regulate that which cannot be convincingly proven.[16] In the United States, there are few or no hard data suggesting that spending money on patients predicted to die alters the availability of resources for other similar patients in the defined population.[17] It is shaky logic to use this nonexistent data in formulating policy on forgoing treatment. It follows then that any prospective determination of futility may be fruit from a poisoned tree. If society gives physicians the authority to determine the nature of futility, it will be on the basis of political and social correctness, not rigorous scientific proof. Is there a higher order to that correctness? The argument could be made that in the absence of convincing proof, maximum treatment for all classifications of illness is fair game. If effectiveness is an unknown quantity, then treating everyone maximally will offer the best chance for capturing the greatest population of those capable of benefit. In such a system, the only patients who can be considered to have treatment failure are those who fail to respond to maximal therapy. Therefore, patients who might die with lesser treatment might not die with more. The only potential limiting factor in such a care plan is the ability to finance it, and that is a political argument, not a medical one. In essence, this argument suggests that the freedom inherent in personal autonomy is exigent enough that every other option should be given a fair shot before that freedom is limited.

In addition, even if it is agreed that intensive care unit (ICU) physicians are in the best position to determine what is medically futile, there is little or no convincing evidence that authorizing physicians to unilaterally determine the nature of futility is a good thing. Physicians, especially those in the United States, do not have a history of bias-free behavior in their dealings with resource allocation.[18] The health care reimbursement system in America promotes and nurtures the provision of ineffective care, by paying for it on the basis of correct paperwork rather than objective evidence of utility. From a business point of view, the American health care system evolved not to treat people but to deliver billable medical services to patients.[19] Management of disease should be an integrated process, to maximize efficiency, minimize cost, and maximize benefit. But because of a historical quirk, physicians normally practice autonomously from hospitals. This arrangement means that decisions with the greatest impact on the institution's costs, quality, and reputation are made by providers who are insensitive to institutional efforts at resource conservation. Methods for reimbursing physicians are separate from methods for reimbursing hospitals. There is potential for physicians enriching themselves by creating demand for expensive services and inducing resource utilization even as the facilities try to minimize the use of such services, to conserve resources.[20]

When medical care was affordable, people paid for it like they paid for groceries. Unexpected medical expenses could be a big financial hit, but it rarely broke anyone. If you really did not need a service, you did not ask for it, because doing so would force you to alter your finances. Health insurance was affordable for the common citizen because it was designed to adequately indemnify him or her against disasters, not pay for health care from the cradle to the grave. The rest was affordable out of pocket. When universal government-sponsored health care in the form of Medicare and Medicaid arrived, personal liability for purchasing and prioritizing health care services vanished and demand escalated, supplied by a burgeoning medical-industrial complex. Physicians were no longer "professionals"; they were "small businesspersons," marketing services to the community instead of hanging out a shingle and waiting to be sought out on the basis of need. The more demand physicians created, the more it was eagerly supplied, and the more the medical-industrial complex prospered. Then the neck of the goose supplying the golden eggs began to stretch. Because the business of medicine as it is practiced by the fee-for-service system rewards resource maximization with no brakes, it was only a matter of time before external moves to control it evolved.

Wennberg[21] warned that business would become extremely important: "Unless the medical profession accepts responsibility for the question of 'which rate [of medical or surgical utilization] is right' and addresses these issues within the current cost-containment context, others will see to it that the 'least is always best' theory dominates by default." Indemnifiers found that it was politically unpopular indeed to suggest cutting back desired services to a public that had been led to believe they were a fundamental right. Political careers could be broken by such decisions. There is nothing so politically powerful as telling constituents things they want to believe. So bureaucrats continued to allow consumers essentially free access to wildly escalating services and insulated themselves from public disfavor by placing providers in harm's way. Indemnifiers effectively conserved resources by simply refusing to pay for services rendered unless providers jumped through administrative hoops.[22] These regulations had a strong bias toward denial when processing claims. Incredibly simple errors ground the process to a halt for weeks or months, creating an incentive for providers to give up and absorb the loss rather than spend the administrative time and money fighting for it. Patients were encouraged to keep using services, but reimbursement to hospitals and providers was cut back by means of "inconvenience blocks." That is, more and more paperwork was required, and if this paperwork was not completed to the letter, the result was nonpayment. Computers were set to deny for the smallest infraction of increasingly complex rules.

It could be argued that the handwriting was on the wall for resource conservation based on benefit defined by consumers with an unlimited incentive to consume. It is impossible to conserve hens if a fox is in charge of the henhouse. But providers quickly reacted to maximize resource accumulation by creatively manipulating the rules. They reacted like constructors of race cars after institution of rule changes designed to slow cars down for safety. Every year, the Indianapolis Motor Speedway promoters make rules to slow the cars down; every year, rules are bent and cars are constructed to go faster. When the dust settled, indemnifiers discovered that the only way to stop efforts to undermine their methods was to institute more novel environments that generated decreasing return for increasing market penetration. Ultimately, these policies evolved to retroactive audits:

resources could be made returnable to indemnifiers if they were found "inappropriate" by some standard 2 or more years after they were expended. Much like the Internal Revenue Service and the Selective Service System, managed care has evolved into a system designed to be bulletproof against external threats its designers knew would be constant.

But none of this accurately addressed the specific problem of futility, and the search continued for a solution. Options other than limitation of care were suggested. Public relations attempts to improve communication with the public regarding the realities of treatments used at the end of life were mounted. The Study to Understand Prognoses and Preferences for Outcomes and Risks of Treatments (SUPPORT)[23] and other studies have been widely recognized as a great source of high-quality data on how end-of-life care is dispensed in the United States. These reports have been disheartening because the understanding between physicians and families of what constitutes futility has been shown to be very shaky, and attempts to improve this discrepancy by improving communication have been largely unsuccessful.[24] Again, the question of whether the problem of resource allocation is severe enough to justify the excision of patient autonomy on the basis of expense has never been satisfactorily answered. Refusing to cover treatment perceived to be futile may be exactly what society should do, but getting the public to agree with this may be too difficult to accomplish without ripping out the core of clinical medicine as we know it. It is simply too early in the game to tell.

The problem of competition for beds dovetails into the broad concept of futility, further complicating it. What is clearly futile treatment for one patient is sometimes fair game for other players in the arena of critical care utilization. These dynamics directly affect the translation of futility to resource utilization in a legal framework. For example, the Von Stetina case[25] involved a previously healthy 27-year-old woman injured in a motor vehicle accident. She was taken to a hospital, where emergency surgery was performed, and she was then admitted to the hospital's ICU. Over the next several days, she seemed to be recovering, but she had been paralyzed and sedated to optimize oxygen transport versus consumption. She accidentally became disconnected from her ventilator, whose alarm had intentionally been turned off, ostensibly to avoid the distraction of false alarms. After she became bradycardic from hypoxemia, the heart rhythm alarm sounded and she was promptly resuscitated. Unfortunately, the cerebral anoxic insult was sufficient to induce a persistent vegetative state, with no hope of recovery.

During the trial for malpractice, it was established that at the time of Von Stetina's admission to the ICU, there were a total of seven patients in the ICU, cared for by three registered nurses and one licensed practical nurse. This staffing was considered to be adequate. However, five more patients were admitted to the unit between midnight and 6 A.M., but the number of nurses remained the same. There was no ICU director in evidence to direct admissions or deal with bed allocation. Accordingly, it was alleged that there were too many patients for the number of nurses present to care for adequately. Ostensibly, Von Stetina's technological hardware failed because her nurse was too busy to observe and monitor her adequately. What were the available nurses busy doing that night? One patient in the ICU at the time of the bed occupancy crisis was close to meeting criteria for brain death, and in fact, the patient was declared dead the next day. Another patient was considered to be in the terminal stages of disease, and that patient died the next day also. It was further established that three other hospitals in the area had vacant beds and a quorum of nurses and could have taken transfers. It was ultimately established that the facility, which held itself to be a critical care unit, did not in fact provide that service, because of staff-to-patient disproportion. The hospital was found liable for a total of $12,470,000. That was more than 20 years ago. The expected settlement for a similar case in the new millennium would be considerably larger.

The Von Stetina case illustrates a resource issue that has yet to be dealt with effectively. Does occupancy of a critical care bed guarantee possession until death or full resolution of the illness for which the patient was admitted? The first-come-first-served "lottery" for ICU beds may make hospitals liable for damages if patients with good prognoses are denied the benefit of critical care resources because nurses are stretched too thin in caring for patients with poor prognoses. There may be a legal obligation to discharge patients with only a borderline possibility of benefiting from intensive care, in order to maintain good standards of care for those patients remaining. If being an early arrival to the ICU does not mean special rights to an ICU bed are granted, then patients deriving marginal benefit from those beds can be moved to make room for those with better prognoses.

As can be gleaned from this discussion, the issue of futility in the ICU is multifactorial and there are few if any clear answers to the perceived problems. Solving some dilemmas creates others. But if the issue is distilled to its essence, at least two tiers for redefining futility at the end of life in critical care float to the surface. First, the notion of futility as being associated only with an end-stage process in which vital signs cannot be supported further is proving to be unworkable, because the consequences of its outcome are larger than the sum of the parts. Moribund patients supported by life-sustaining machinery in an ICU assume a thin veneer of life, but underneath there is only an inanimate shell. The cost to support these patients is disproportionally high compared with the cost of other health care and is unfairly borne by a tax base that has no say in allocation. Society needs to consider new definitions of futility at the end of life that take into account fallacious appearances of viability. Society needs options that more accurately sensitize the concept of futility to the realities of its clinical consequences. It must be permissible to say that futile treatment is treatment given to a patient who is not medically viable. Under the current futility rules, there is a strong incentive to treat on the basis of unrealistic expectation and there is too little liability if the patient being treated persists in unrealistic care plans. There is no balance of power between these forces.

But if this argument is rejected on the grounds that no one has convincingly proven that finances matter in the grand scheme, and that maximizing care for all comers generates a marginally improved outcome, even for a diminishing population, there is another possible argument for redefining futility. Sustaining vital signs in the face of multiple organ system failure causes profound and unrelenting discomfort. The decision to limit futile care results not just in financial savings but in improved patient comfort during the dying process. There is a plethora of evidence that maintenance of moribund but awake patients on dead-end life support is uncomfortable and that the need to provide sedation regimens to ameliorate this discomfort destroys the chance for any positive quality of life.

Before the technological revolution in critical care medicine, agitation and discomfort were relatively minor issues. Little could be done for critically ill patients beyond making them as comfortable as possible and observing them for treatable decompensations. Modern ICUs now have the potential to sustain organ system failure, but at the cost of pinning the patient firmly to the bed, with tubes and appliances in every orifice, resulting in disquietude and discomfort.[26] Physical discomfort plus distorted and interrupted metabolic homeostasis, endocrine insufficiency, acute and chronic cardiopulmonary decompensations, poor tissue perfusion, polypharmacy, and disruption of the sleep–wake cycle due to immobilization cause varying degrees of "brain failure."[27] Brain failure is just as relevant as renal or hepatic failure and produces profound discomfort that is difficult or impossible to ameliorate without chemical and physical restraint.

The intensive care environment is a repository for stress factors of a hemodynamic and metabolic nature.[28] Stress usually produces a heightened sense of fear and anxiety, which causes increased norepinephrine turnover in the limbic regions (hippocampus, amygdala, locus coeruleus) and cerebral cortex. Panic attacks, insomnia, accentuated startle, autonomic hyperarousal, and hypervigilance are characteristics of noradrenergic hyperfunction. The limbic and cortical regions innervated by the locus coeruleus are thought to be involved in the elaboration of adaptive responses to stress. Animals that have experienced stress in the past and find themselves in the environment in which the stress was previously produced show increased responsiveness to excitatory stimuli previously experienced. Limited exposure to stress that does not increase noradrenergic activity in control animals increases norepinephrine release in animals previously exposed to the same kind of stress. Dopaminergic enervation of the medial and dorsolateral prefrontal cortex appears to be particularly vulnerable to repetitive stress. In sensitized persons, relatively low levels of stress may promote significant responses such as anxiety, panic, hypervigilance, exaggerated startle reflexes, and paranoia.

The acute behavioral responses can be brought about by the activation of neurotransmission-modulated humoral factors resulting from psychological and physical trauma. These represent evolutionary adaptive responses critical for survival in an uncertain and potentially dangerous environment. These compensatory responses were presumably created at a time in the universe when there were no high-tech surrogates for naturally induced environmental stress. The highly stressful environment of the ICU leads to loss of orientation to time and place. Monotonous sensory input (e.g., from repetitive and noisy monitoring equipment), prolonged immo-bilization (especially with indwelling life-support hardware), frequently interrupted sleep patterns, and social isolation eventually contribute to the onset of brain dysfunction. Patients in the hybrid intensive care environment undergo stress but no natural environmental threat, so the response not only is wasted but becomes an open-ended detriment. Conditioned fear and recollection of immobilization stress may be experienced by patients who have undergone traumatic emergency endotracheal intubation and mechan-ical ventilation in the past. In ICU patients, the sensitizing factor may result from hemodynamic and metabolic decompensations as a result of multiple system insufficiency. Behavioral sensitization to stress may also involve "memory imprinting" alterations in noradrenergic function. This is thought to be the mechanism of posttraumatic stress disorder, which was originally recognized in Vietnam veterans but is now recognized as a sequela of other prolonged, inordinately stressful events, as in the case of a patient with an unpleasant ICU history who enters unexpected delirium quickly after a subsequent admission.[29]

Delirium resulting from dopaminergic hyperfunction is characterized by global disorders of cognition and wakefulness and by impairment of psychomotor behavior.[30] Major cognitive functions such as perception, deductive reasoning, memory, attention, and orientation are globally disordered. Excessive motor activity frequently accompanies severe cases of delirium. When this occurs, the resulting constellation of symptoms is called agitated delirium. This syndrome is not uncommon after extremely stressful ICU stays, especially if the patient experienced untreated pain, anxiety, or delirium during a previous admission.

Therefore, normally beneficial responses act to the patient's detriment in the artificial, intensive care environment, and the only practical way to block them is to dull them with central nervous system–depressing medication, which in turn blocks the patient's view and experience of his or her world.

The current definition of futility (the inability to sustain vital signs in a warm cadaver) in fact perpetuates global and multilevel discomfort for helpless patients who can neither communicate their discomfort nor make it stop. They must be sedated to give the appearance of comfort. Making an argument of limiting "futile" care just to save money suggests an interest in skimping on the basis of a prioritization concept not universally accepted. To do so prompts criticism, particularly from minorities and disabled individuals. If "medically inappropriate" care causes pain, suffering, and discomfort, then the money issue, if it exists, is not relevant. Life support for patients predicted to die does not equal comfort care, and "medically appropriate" care, supported by literature on evidence-based medicine, results in "better" care of patients at the end of life. Is the argument for futility a money issue or a patient-comfort issue? If it is a money issue, time will tell who is willing to continue underwriting futile care. If it is a patient-comfort issue, it is unreasonable to force physicians to go against their expert judgment when families insist on maintaining prolonged discomfort for reasons that are defensible only in emotional terms.

Health care consumers normally consult physicians for problems they cannot resolve on their own. A surgical consultation does not guarantee a surgical procedure. It generates an opinion regarding whether surgical intervention might be beneficial, and the surgeon is never mandated to perform surgery simply because the patient desires it. However, it seems that critical care physicians cannot act on any clinical judgment with regard to futility if that judgment is not acceptable to family surrogates. Futility can (and should) be defined in terms of failure of organ systems, and organ system failure can be extrapolated to include human discomfort. If futility is defined in terms of the number of failed organ systems, the length of such failures, and the number of life-support machines needed to maintain viability, ICU physicians then derive more support from the peer-reviewed literature on evidence-based medicine to bolster their prognostications. Dismal predictions of future viability for these kinds of patients are very accurate in the peer-reviewed medical literature. And this authority increases its enforceability. The prospect of maintaining discomfort is difficult to defend on the basis of irrational hope. If patients and their surrogates are granted unlimited authority, scarce resources will be used to warehouse increasing numbers of warm cadavers. In an economy seeking to maximize use of scarce resources, how far should society support the autonomy of groups who have an incentive to maximize expenditures of others to support their own ends? How much is society willing to pay for unlimited patient autonomy?

References

[1]Wu AW, Damiano AM, Lynn J, et al: Predicting future functional status for seriously ill hospitalized adults. The SUPPORT prognostic model. Ann Intern Med 1995;122:342–50.

[2]Crippen D: Critical care and the Internet. A clinician's perspective. Crit Care Clin 1999;15:605–14, vii.

[3]Hiatt HH: Protecting the medical commons: who is responsible? N Engl J Med 1975;293:235–41.

[4]Berenson RA: Intensive Care Units (ICUs): Clinical Outcomes, Costs and Decisionmaking (Health Technology Case Study 28). Washington, DC: Office of Technology Assessment, 1984.

[5]Engelhardt HT Jr, Rie MA: Intensive care units, scarce resources, and conflicting principles of justice. JAMA 1986;255:1159–64.

[6]H.J. RES 29. March 6, 2001.

[7]A controlled trial to improve care for seriously ill hospitalized patients. The Study to Understand Prognoses and Preferences for Outcomes and Risks of Treatments (SUPPORT). The SUPPORT Principal Investigators. JAMA 1995;274:1591–8.

[8]Wanzer SH, Adelstein SJ, Cranford RE, et al: The physician's responsibility toward hopelessly ill patients. N Engl J Med 1984;310:955–9.

[9]Chelluri L, Pinsky MR, Donahoe MP, et al: Long-term outcome of critically ill elderly patients requiring intensive care. JAMA 1993;269:3119–23.

[10]Knaus WA, Draper EA, Wagner DP, et al: Prognosis in acute organ-system failure. Ann Surg 1985;202:685–93.

[11]Breen CM, Abernethy AP, Abbott KH, et al: Conflict associated with decisions to limit life-sustaining treatment in intensive care units. J Gen Intern Med 2001;16:283–9.

[12]Wenger NS, Kanouse DE, Collins RL, et al: End-of-life discussions and preferences among persons with HIV. JAMA 2001;285:2880–7.

[13]Field BE, Devich LE, Carlson RW: Impact of a comprehensive supportive care team on management of hopelessly ill patients with multiple organ failure. Chest 1989;96:353–6.

[14]Burrows R: Removal of life support in intensive care units. Med Law 1994;13:489–500.

[15]Francis LP: Legal rights to health care at the end of life. JAMA 1999;282:2079.

[16]Consensus statement of the Society of Critical Care Medicine's Ethics Committee regarding futile and other possibly inadvisable treatments. Crit Care Med 1997;25:887–91.

[17]Pronovost P, Angus DC: Economics of end-of-life care in the intensive care unit. Crit Care

Med 2001;29:N46–51.

[18]Taylor M: Investigation heats up. Probe of alleged kickbacks at Tenet hospitals escalates. Mod Healthc 2001;31:20–1.

[19]Kleinke JD: Bleeding Edge: The Business of Health Care Delivery in the New Century. Gaithersburg, MD: Aspen, 1998.

[20]Daniels N: Why saying no to patients in the United States is so hard. Cost containment, justice, and provider autonomy. N Engl J Med 1986;314:1380–3.

[21]Wennberg J: The paradox of appropriate care. JAMA 1987;258:2568–9.

[22]Grumet GW: Health care rationing through inconvenience. The third party's secret weapon. N Engl J Med 1989;321:607–11.

[23]Lynn J, Teno JM, Phillips RS, et al: Perceptions by family members of the dying experience of older and seriously ill patients. SUPPORT Investigators. Study to Understand Prognoses and Preferences for Outcomes and Risks of Treatments. Ann Intern Med 1997;126:97–106.

[24]Marbella AM, Desbiens NA, Mueller-Rizner N, et al: Surrogates' agreement with patients' resuscitation preferences: effect of age, relationship, and SUPPORT intervention. Study to Understand Prognoses and Preferences for Outcomes and Risks of Treatment. J Crit Care 1998;13:140–5.

[25]Von Stetina vs Florida Medical Center. Florida Law Weekly. May 24, 1985.

[26]Crippen D: Agitation in the ICU, part one: anatomical and physiologic basis for the agitated state. Crit Care 1999;3:R35–46.

[27]Crippen D: Understanding the neurohumoral causes of anxiety in the ICU. Clinical consequences include agitation, brain failure, delirium. J Crit Illn 1995;10:550–5, 559–60.

[28]Crippen DW: Neurologic monitoring in the intensive care unit. New Horiz 1994;2:107–20.

[29]Scragg P, Jones A, Fauvel N: Psychological problems following ICU treatment. Anaesthesia 2001;56:9–14.

[30]Crippen D: Life-threatening brain failure and agitation in the intensive care unit. Crit Care 2000;4:81–90.

Discussion of the
Ethical Aspects of Futility

David F. Kelly, PhD

In this concluding section I will not repeat the points I made earlier in the book, though I will refer to them. I am not clinically trained. I am not a physician or a nurse. Thus I cannot be sure that the cases were properly and unambiguously designed. Perhaps there is a valid medical basis for the varying prognoses and treatment options. I am not able to make medical comments on what the various doctors would do. But I can put myself in the position of the many patients and families who request the ethics consultations in which I and my students take part. The patients may have gotten, or may think they have gotten, different prognoses and different treatment options from the different doctors who examined them. I think this problem is most apparent in the case of Patient A and so I will start there.

Patient A

Treatment for Patient A is clearly not in any sense medically futile as I previously defined it. Patient A is presented at the beginning of the book as "a critically ill and unstable patient who is predicted to benefit from short-term critical care. He receives aggressive care with a strong potential to reverse organ system insufficiency and enable him to become a productive member of society once more." Thus if I understand his situation correctly, there is a very good chance that he can be fixed, at least after it is determined that he might "respond neurologically to salvage treatment," as Dr. Batchelor in the United Kingdom puts it. Patient A surely wants to be near a hospital with the equipment, talent, and willingness to fix him. Dr. Fisher in Australia, Dr. van der Spoel in the Netherlands, Dr. Tan in China, Dr. Roy-Shapira in Israel, and Dr. Chalfin in the United States would admit him and treat him, though with some possibly important differences in available resources. Dr. Batchelor, Dr. Kapadia in India, and Dr. Streat in New Zealand would admit him and treat him in their intensive care units (ICUs) but only after assurance of "a realistic chance of brain recovery," as

Dr. Kapadia notes. Dr. Streat writes that his hospital calls it "admission with reservations." Only Dr. Burrows in South Africa would not admit Patient A to his ICU.

I repeat that I cannot claim to know that the case with its clinical details is unambiguous. I do know that it was created by practicing critical care physicians in the United States to present a very sick patient whose cure could reasonably be achieved. The book's editors assumed that intensive care physicians would want to try to save him. We recognized of course that some nations would not have the resources to treat him that were available to others. But we at least assumed that all physicians would say that if they had unlimited resources, they would treat him and probably fix him. Yet Dr. Burrows from South Africa says that he would not let him in even if his hospital had unlimited resources. Burrows tells us that "the prognosis is grim, and the probability of death under these circumstances is extremely high." He continues:

> To ask what one would do supposing resources were infinite implies that more and more resources should be expended on those with a vanishingly small chance of survival. However, should the patient or relatives wish to continue treatment under these circumstances, there does not seem to be any point (short of decomposition) at which the physician may insist on stopping treatment.

What is going on here? I cannot be certain, but I suspect two dynamics. First, because medicine is an art and not an exact science, doctors often differ about prognoses. Perhaps Patient A's case is not as clear as we thought when we created it. Second, perhaps there is something societal going on, the kind of social cohesion that earlier in this book I suggested is lacking in the United States. I want to spend some time on each of these possibilities.

First, different prognoses. The clinical bioethicist learns quickly the importance of communication in a fast-paced American hospital. He or she also learns how common it is that no one really understands. In the graduate heath care ethics programs that I direct and teach in at Duquesne University in Pittsburgh, Pennsylvania, all students are required to take a course in health care communication ethics. Dr. Pat Arneson, whose field of expertise is health communication, tries to give future ethicists some knowledge of and training in how health care institutions make communication hard and how the many differently trained and educated health care professionals find it difficult to talk to each other and to patients and families. Actual practice as a clinical ethicist has taught me that you can never presume that people actually understand anything until you get them together and have them speak to each other. Even then, of course, there is sometimes refusal or inability to understand. Some families simply cannot or will not accept even the clearest prognosis after all the doctors and nurses involved have made it quite clear to them. Grief or guilt or anger or simple stubbornness sometimes weakens or even destroys communication.

But I have also found that many times the problem does not lie only with the patients or families. It lies also with the pace of intensive medicine. In his examination of the clinical approaches to Patient C by the 11 intensivists, Dr. Levy insists that this is often the case. Sometimes doctors have never really tried to communicate. In other cases the medical chart is inconsistent: neurological consultations differ about stroke sequelae, cardiologists differ about the severity of an insult, the lung doctor is optimistic and the kidney doctor sees no hope, one nurse claims the patient is awake and alert and another claims he is comatose. I have even been involved with a case in which a physician charted the patient as brain-dead even though she responded to simple stimuli. Now sometimes this means bad medicine. But sometimes it means only that the various opinions have been given at different times and with different medications. Or it may mean simply that medicine is an art, not an exact science. Some diagnoses are hard to make. Dr. Burrows himself points this out: "Prognostication at the end of life is notoriously uncertain."

The bottom line here is that patients and (more usually in the ICU) patients' families have to make decisions without the kind of information they think they need. Patient A's South African family will probably be told that he has little or no hope, though Dr. Burrows does say that wealthy families would be offered the possibility of a transfer to another institution. Patient A's American family will be given every assurance that the ICU will fix him. And the problem of medical futility emerges in this kind of context. Over and over, medical studies have shown the difficulty of basing sure diagnoses on easily quantified clinical data. As Dr. Kilcullen notes in his discussion of Patient A's case and treatment, various scales of morbidity have been tried, and although they are surely helpful, they fail to predict death with accuracy. As I noted, there are always cases in which patients have survived and even thrived against all odds. Families want this for their own loved ones, too.

I can offer one suggestion for those of us who work with very sick patients and their families. What families want to know above all is, what is the best possible outcome? In ethics consultations, we ask that question of doctors over and over again. If the antibiotics cure her sepsis, if the heparin stops the strokes, if the vasopressors stabilize her blood pressure and the dialysis gets her over the acute kidney failure, and if her brain comes back from the bilateral occipital anoxia as much as you can reasonably hope it might, what will she be like? Will she be blind and dumb? Will she walk? How? Will she recognize anyone? Will she be able to eat ice cream? Watch TV? Hug her grandchildren? It is amazing to me how often families have not been given the answers to these questions. Usually they understand if the doctor says it is too early to know. But they need to be told what the doctors think about prognosis for the whole person. And they need to be told early and every day. Intensive care units (and hospital floors, for that matter) need family coordinators—nurses whose job it is to keep current with the case and talk to the family, to set up conferences with the physicians to keep the family abreast of what is happening and what is likely to happen. I do not claim that this approach will eliminate cases in which families insist on treating even patients like Patient C. But my experience suggests that it often allows families to understand that now is the time to stop and allow death to happen.

The second thought I have about Patient A and his differing situation among the responding physicians—most would treat him, but some would be at least hesitant, and in Dr. Burrows' hospital he would not even be admitted to the ICU—is that this clearly points to societal agreements that differ among nations. Dr. Burrows' response suggests that he may respond as he does not because he thinks that nowhere can critical care save and fix this patient but because he thinks that in his hospital in South Africa, it would be wrong to try. "It is unconscionable that in a country where human immunodeficiency virus (HIV) infection is epidemic, such funds are used for those whose chance of survival is remote." And that is a different issue altogether.

I will begin here by saying that in my judgment, it is unethical to confuse these two issues when dealing with patients and their families. If Patient A can indeed be treated and cured but will not be treated because of resource constraints (the monies and energies are ethically better spent on patients with HIV or acquired immunodeficiency syndrome or on fighting malnutrition or diarrhea), it is still wrong to tell him and members of his family that there is nothing that can be done. Honesty requires that they be told that a cure is possible but that the means for achieving that cure are not available here and now because social decisions have been made to allocate resources differently.

This approach is important for a number of reasons, not all of them deontological, to use philosophers' language for an a priori–based obligation that ought to be followed regardless of consequences. Yes, deontologically the obligation of truth-telling ought to compel one, in at least most situations, to tell the truth and not escape the easy way. The patient's team ought to tell the truth here even though it is far easier just to tell the family that Patient A has no hope of a cure and let the family infer from this that the team means he is medically incurable, whereas what is really meant is that he is financially incurable. (This kind of trick, by the way, was for a long time permitted in Catholic medical ethics under the rubric of "strict mental reservation," a device no one to my knowledge now uses in medical ethics, Catholic or not.)

But there are consequential reasons as well. In the immediate sense, it may be the case that the family will have the resources to move the patient elsewhere, as Dr. Burrows recognizes, or to fight the system and get curative treatment. But for me, it is in the larger social sense that truth-telling here is most important. It is only if people start to understand the kinds of allocation that really do occur—and this not only in the developing world but also in developed countries, such as the United States—that social understanding will allow public investigation and possible change. In the United States, for example, if a primary care physician tells an uninsured person that he or she is not accepting new patients, whereas he or she really is accepting insured patients, the physician encourages ignorance of an unethical health care system. So the doctor who cannot treat a patient because of scarce resources has, I think, an obligation to tell the truth about that reason.

Different countries have different implicit and explicit social agreements. But all nations, even the United States, as Dr. Gipe points out, have to ration somehow. Some health systems, for example, have explicit rules that deny certain treatments to persons above a certain age. Others have implicit understandings that patients whose cure costs "too much" will not be admitted to the ICU. These implicit agreements are likely to be embedded in that nation's medical standard of care without ever being explicitly articulated. There are dangers with both of these approaches, of course. Explicit regulation may be motivated more by political interests or special interest lobbying than by ethical concerns of access and fair distribution. Implicit understandings are even more problematic, for they are open to different interpretation by different physicians and are terribly hard to examine.

Thus, social agreements about allocation of health care resources— and, by the way, about macro-allocation of resources to health care—can be explicit or implicit. Usually there is some messy combination of the two.

Theoretically, explicit allocation is best. But it is exquisitely hard to accomplish. How can you defend a decision not to treat patients curable only at enormous cost? Where exactly do you draw the line? So governments hide behind slogans. In the United States, the slogan might be something about freedom from governmental interference, freedom of choice of doctors, the greatness of American competition, the evil of socialist systems like those in Britain and Canada, and so on, whereas the reality is lack of access, overutilization of emergency departments for common ailments by people rejected from primary care, tens of millions uninsured, and busloads of elderly people going *to* Canada for their prescription drugs so that they do not have to choose between needed medication and food on the table. All countries have social agreements of some kind. And they differ from one another.

But there is no a priori philosophical reason to reject rationing schemes as inherently unjust. In the United States, the health care system rations implicitly all the time, primarily by denying access to the poor and the near poor, and explicitly in some insurance contracts and most famously in the Oregon Medicaid allocation plan that proposes a cutoff point on a list of treatments. I happen to think that America's discrimination against the poor is unjust, that some of the insurance contracts are unjust, and that the Oregon Plan is perhaps as close to just as one is going to get, though there are still serious problems with it both as process and as outcome. But allocation schemes that discriminate justly—that rightly propose that certain treatments not be paid for by a national health insurance because the nation's wealth is better spent elsewhere—are just.

Thus in comparing the varying responses to Patient A, I find the range of approaches I have noted. Some of the physicians would admit and treat and probably fix. Others would admit with hesitation, or only after investigation, or with some sort of administrative protocol. One would not admit at all. Most would look primarily or perhaps only at Patient A himself; others would take the general welfare and common good of others in the nation into account. These differences stem from different implicit and explicit social agreements. These in turn are why in some parts of the world one simply does not expect access to multiple organ transplantations or to extremely expensive neonatal support for infants born at a gestational age of 22 weeks, whereas in other nations these treatments are available and expected (at least in the case of those with insurance).

Whether the implicit and explicit cost-containment schemes that seem to be at work in the responses of some of the doctors, especially Dr. Burrows, to Patient A are just is a question I cannot answer. It depends on too many factors: national wealth, the kind of basic health care system in place, the kind of government that makes the rules, whether costly treatment is justly denied (no one over age x or with condition y will receive a heart transplant) or unjustly denied (no one of a certain race or tribe or political party or no one without connections in high places will receive the transplant). Details like these determine the moral quality of the allocation scheme. But on the face of it, Dr. Burrows' argument, amplified in his overview of proposed treatment approaches to Patient C, that health care resources ought to go to the many and not the very few is compelling. In any case, such social agreements are not necessarily morally wrong; there is no a priori basis for claiming they are.

But there is one more important issue here, one that Dr. Hoyt brings up in his analysis of Patient A's case. Is it up to the individual physician to make this kind of decision, to decide that justice in allocating resources is a reason for refusing admittance to a patient for whom very costly treatment might be truly beneficial? It is at best risky and quite possibly unjust for that to be the process. Even such a thoroughgoing utilitarian as Peter Singer, known for his insistence that resources be distributed globally so that they might do the most good, argued that "the physician should not also be the person who decides which forms of health care are sufficiently cost-effective to be offered to her or his patient. Leaving this decision to the physician may clash too violently with the principle that physicians should further the best interests of their patients."[1] Such rationing schemes are better debated in public, enacted by public legislation or regulation, and left open to some sort of public critique and amendment. In any case, these are *not* medical decisions. Treatment for Patient A (at least, assuming the findings of the neurological evaluation are hopeful) may in no way be called medically futile. He can be fixed. These decisions are thus social, economic, political, and ethical decisions. They are far better made publicly than privately. And they ought never to be defended as if they were made on the basis of medical expertise.

Nonetheless, I cannot conclude that physicians always act unethically when they reject costly treatment for their patients. As I have noted, even implicit rationing schemes may be just. They may be based on a social understanding within a country whereby all agree, albeit implicitly, that costly treatment protocols are simply beyond the capability of that nation's medical system if basic care is to be given to all citizens. Physicians who act in accordance with such an understanding cannot be said to act unethically. Indeed, perhaps that nation has made its judgments about such matters better than the United States has done. Or, of course, perhaps not. It is simply not possible to say without conducting an extensive investigation of a nation's health care system.

I will conclude this section by noting the particular importance of some of the points made by Dr. Kilcullen in his comments on Patient A's case. He is absolutely right when he says that whereas in the United States, families have veto power over physicians' decisions to stop treatment, "families elsewhere in the world possess no such veto power." I argued earlier in the book that physicians cannot claim that treating patients like Patient A is medically futile. They ought not to unilaterally claim, on the basis of medical expertise, that treatment is useless. But I did not state that refusal to treat is unjust. Although in the present American system it appears on the basis of case precedent (see, for example, *In re Helga Wanglie*)[2] to be illegal, and although it would be wrong for individual critical care physicians to refuse to treat Patient A, even if they did so on the grounds of the need for a just allocation of resources, the United States and other wealthy nations are not required to treat Patient A if they arrive at this agreement after a discussion of the ethical issues involved in the case and conclude and announce publicly that Patient A's treatment is simply too costly to afford. I even suggested that such policies, if made publicly by individual hospitals, would not be unethical, although it is very likely that they would be challenged in court.

In any case, the basic argument Dr. Kilcullen makes that at some point even rich nations like the United States will have to face answering the question about treating even curable patients like Patient A is entirely correct. The United States may decide that treatment of the patient will continue. And that may be the right decision. As a potential Patient A, from the perspective of my own self-interest, I hope so. But it may also be the wrong decision ethically. It may be unjust to cure Patient A while millions in America lack basic access to primary care. Or it may be that in the United States, both ought to be done. But then what about malnutrition in Africa? Is spending money on Patient A (or on opera and professional football) just while millions starve? Dr. Douglas puts it this way: "There is a glaring and contradicting irony between caring for terminally ill elderly patients using physiologically futile therapeutic interventions, in developed societies, and providing any level of critical care in developing countries. . . . a pervasive lack of minimal housing, sewerage, and access to clean drinking water outweighs the philosophical debate being discussed here." I would rather insist that these issues are and must be a part of that debate. Getting at answers to these questions is exquisitely difficult. But, as Drs. Douglas and Kilcullen forcefully state, they must be asked.

Patients B and C

I will discuss Patients B and C together. Here the question of medical futility can reasonably be said to arise.

Patient B is described as

> a critically ill patient who may or may not benefit from the application of critical care technology and who is treated aggressively. Subsequently, he stops benefiting from treatment and becomes dependent on life support. A critical deadlock is reached: the patient's family desires to maintain life-support systems indefinitely, with negligible predicted benefit, and physicians desire to stop the same care because it will not return the patient to sentient life.

And Patient C is described as

> a moribund patient with multiple organ system failure who desires the use of life-support systems despite the expressed opinion of critical care physicians that such care will do nothing but increase his discomfort during the inevitable dying process.

I repeat that as an ethicist who is not a physician, I cannot say that the cases were perfectly drawn to exhibit these characteristics. But Patient C—from the beginning—and Patient B—at a later point in his progressive deterioration—are both cases where medical futility might reasonably be claimed. The question here must be whether it is right to claim it.

Let me begin here with my own judgment regarding whether treatment for Patients B and C may rightly be called medically futile. In the case of Patient B, if I understand it correctly, the answer is no. Patient B's family correctly claim that life-sustaining treatment will keep him alive. So the treatment is not, in the restrictive meaning that I claim the term must have, medically futile. It is morally extraordinary and it is, as some contributors to this book have suggested, medically inappropriate given the certainly grim prognosis. I would very much like the United States to arrive at the conclusion that Patient B should not be treated. I would like hospitals to announce publicly that they will not keep people like him alive. They should do this, again quite publicly, on the basis of social justice and the proper allocation of scarce resources. But I do not think it correct to claim that this is a specifically medical decision lacking in any social, ethical, or political dimensions such that only physicians have the expertise to make the decision (and thus the physician must unilaterally refuse to treat).

Let me present a debate in Roman Catholic medical ethics that might serve to clarify why I say this. The tradition of Catholic medical ethics has been quite flexible about the issue of forgoing treatment. Treatments can be determined to be morally extraordinary, and thus optional, for a number of reasons. It comes down to a balancing of benefits and burdens. And financial exigency can be considered; indeed, most of today's Catholic ethicists would say that it *must* be considered. Thus life-sustaining treatment for Patient B is morally extraordinary; indeed, I would argue that it is stupid. It is also, I think, unjust, but the injustice is a systemic injustice that does not necessarily give the individual physician the right to choose to refuse to administer life-sustaining treatment in order to correct it.

Now there are some ethicists and not a few American Catholic bishops who claim that it is morally obligatory to use tube feedings for patients in a persistent vegetative state (PVS). They have argued that tube feeding is a not medical treatment but that it is human care and always obligatory (except when the patient cannot absorb the nutrition or when it will cause discomfort, which is not the case with PVS patients). They have even claimed that to withdraw tube feeding from PVS patients is to kill them, that it is active euthanasia. Now, I am convinced that those who make this claim misunderstand their own tradition. And indeed, other Catholic medical ethicists and other American bishops have said this. To withhold or withdraw tube feeding from PVS patients is not to kill them, but it is, like the withdrawal of a ventilator, the forgoing of morally extraordinary means of keeping them alive. The recent *Ethical and Religious Directives for Catholic Health Care Services*[3] has said as much; at least, it says that this is one acceptable approach to the issue.

But the very fact that there is such a debate shows that ethicists and religious leaders differ about the *value* of tube feeding in PVS patients. They do not differ about the outcome, assuming of course that the diagnosis has been properly made, which is not always the case. They do not claim that the patient will wake up. They claim that feeding is of human value even in this context. I think they are wrong. But that judgment of mine is not a medical judgment. It is a moral one, based on my own life experience, values, reasoning, and so on. Now, I am not being a relativist here. I think I am right and they are wrong. But I do not think that our disagreement is based on different medical expertise. Hence life-sustaining treatment for Patient B cannot be said to be medically futile.

None of this means, of course, that society (public funds) is obliged to pay for Patient B's treatment. I would applaud a public decision in the United States by Medicare and Medicaid to refuse to insure PVS patients, unlikely though this is in the current American political context. I would applaud a hospital or a nursing home that announced publicly that it had, after public ethical discussion, decided to treat PVS patients only if all costs were covered by private sources, or even that it had decided that its own limitations meant it could not treat PVS patients at all and still treat others, regardless of full payment. Here, too, there is virtually no chance of any health care institution actually doing this in the current American health care ethos. But to do so would be just.

Nonetheless, life-sustaining treatment in Patient B's case is not medically futile.

Patient C, on the other hand, may well be different. If it is indeed the case that Patient C's life cannot be extended by a reasonably significant period—and I have suggested that anything less than 2 or 3 days would not count as a significant extension and that 2 weeks or more would be significant—then life-sustaining treatment for Patient C is indeed medically futile, and physicians must not offer him such treatment. I really do not know where the line can be drawn between 3 days and 2 weeks. And some may reasonably differ even about these limits. These are moral decisions and they do not lend themselves to quantitative certainty. I am not pleased with that, but I do not know how to do better.

This does not, of course, mean that Patient C should be treated even if the ICU could keep him alive for months. The same implicit and explicit societal agreements that may justly and rightly apply to Patient A clearly apply to both Patient B and Patient C. Nations that hesitate to treat Patient A will be even more hesitant about treating Patients B and C. And that is, of course, what the responses of the 11 intensivists suggest.

Dr. Burrows in South Africa would, consistent with his decision for Patient A, not treat either Patient B or Patient C. In Australia, Dr. Fisher might treat Patient B for a short period while he tried to convince the family members to change their minds. If they did not, he would try to get other opinions or to transfer Patient B to another ICU. This approach is consistent with the American legal understanding of medical futility, patient autonomy, and surrogate authority. He might offer some simple treatments to Patient C, but not more.

Regarding Patient B, Dr. Batchelor in the United Kingdom states: "One of the basic tenets of ethics is to do no harm. Admission to an ICU would prolong this man's dying but not his life. . . . It is my feeling that intensive care for Patient B would be cruel and inhumane treatment." Now, this adds an essential dimension that is almost always overlooked. But there is one further point here. Why should the end-of-life treatment for Patient B in an ICU be cruel and unusual? What about sedation? Dr. Crippen notes: "There is a plethora of evidence that maintenance of moribund but awake patients on dead-end life support is uncomfortable and that the need to provide sedation regimens to ameliorate this discomfort destroys the chance for any positive quality of life." And there's the rub. One gets back into quality of life, which means getting back into value judgments, which means getting back to where one started. Patients might choose to be kept sedated and alive. People might say in their advance directives that they do indeed want feeding tubes if they are ever be in a PVS, despite the fact that their quality of life would be absolutely zero. I have noted that some American Catholic moralists and bishops say exactly that (though perhaps without admitting the zero). These patients and these surrogates and these moralists and these bishops are wrong. But the decision not to treat Patient B has to be made for reasons other than purely medical ones; life-sustaining treatment for Patient B, if I understand the case correctly, is not medically futile. With regard to Patient C, Dr. Batchelor says that he would almost certainly never get to her ICU in the first place.

Dr. Kapadia in India would treat Patient B, though there would be an attempt to transfer him to another institution. But Dr. Kapadia repeats what he said about Patient A. The hospital would treat and would bear the expense. Dr. Kapadia goes on, however, to speak about his communication with the family. He says: "In rare cases, the family might insist that we do everything. I often view this as a failure of communication on my part. . . . Not infrequently, the situation is that the patient, an elderly individual, has family in a wealthier part of the world, usually the United States, and because of cultural differences or maybe guilt, the family wants everything done." Precisely. Social agreements differ. Communication is essential. Dr. Kapadia would try very hard not to admit Patient C, but as I understand it, Patient C's "primary consultant" would have the right to insist on ICU admission. Even then, however, Dr. Kapadia would try to limit treatment.

In New Zealand, Dr. Streat would not admit either Patient B or Patient C. Relative to Patient C he says: "As with the first two cases, Patient C's case is simply unrealistic in New Zealand. . . . with regard to the statement 'When options are read to him, he desires them all,' no 'options' would be read to him." Now this is proper for Patient C, I think, though only under the assumption that life-sustaining treatment is indeed medically futile, which it may well be. But Dr. Streat implies that this applies also to Patients A and B ("As with the first two cases"). I am not sure how this applies to Patient A, given that Dr. Streat has said that he would admit Patient A if his neurological deficit shows hope for recovery. Relative to Patient B, however, at least from the American legal and ethical perspective, failure to offer options would be paternalism. The physician should explain that there are treatments that could keep Patient B alive but that because of a general social decision to allocate resources more justly, these treatments are never offered in New Zealand. It is possible, of course, that the social agreement is generally known and quite public, so that a physician's refusal to offer life-sustaining treatment is widely understood as being an ethically right social decision and not just a medical decision.

Dr. van der Spoel in the Netherlands and Dr. Tan in Hong Kong would not admit either Patient B or Patient C. In Russia, Dr. Karakozov would treat Patient B, but he admits that Patient B would get care only if he has insurance or powerful relatives. He notes that "under the newly adopted laws in Russia, people have the right to insist on any kind of treatment that is available through the local hospital" but that more than this requires insurance or wealth or connections. He also notes that paternalism is still common, that patients "usually believe what the doctor says." If Patient B did arrive at his ICU, he would probably treat him: "I realize that all this treatment might be futile and expensive, but I would be unable to resist the temptation to try it." It may be that Russia is going through something akin to what American medicine went through after World War II, when doctors often tried to do everything to keep patients alive and when one of the motives was to gain experience with the new techniques. But this is only a first guess. Further comment would require a thorough knowledge of health care culture and of how it is adapting to the seismic change from the Soviet system. And in the United States as well, wealth and insurance and connections are too often the keys to access.

In Israel, Dr. Roy-Shapira would not treat Patient B. He notes that there are three reasons to stop medical treatment: first, if the patient refuses it; second, if allocation of resources requires that treatment be stopped; and third, if medical treatment is not indicated. He correctly notes that when treatment is forgone for allocation reasons, "this is not a medical question but a political or social question." He claims as well that "in Patient B's case, . . . treatment would only prolong death and thus would do more harm than good. When medical care is not indicated, neither the wishes of the patient nor those of his relatives are relevant. This is a technical issue, and it is the decision of the physician alone." This is, of course, the very essence of medical futility. For reasons I have already enunciated, I disagree with him when he says that this applies to Patient B. But he is quite right, I think, when he goes on to say that when treatment *is* what I have called medically futile, it is "cruel to ask family members." And the example he adds is indeed an example of strict medical futility: "It is not paternalistic to refuse to prescribe antibiotics for the common cold, regardless of the patient's wishes, and it is not paternalistic to refuse to operate when the risk of the operation outweighs the possible benefits." Quite right (although life-sustaining treatment that prolongs life differs ethically from both of these examples). "Similarly," he goes on, "it is not paternalistic to stop treatment when it can no longer accomplish its goals." This, I have argued, depends on what kinds of goals it cannot accomplish.

Interestingly, Dr. Roy-Shapira is alone in saying that treatment for Patient C cannot initially be ruled out. "It is possible that simple measures . . . would return him to his premorbid state." Here again I cannot be certain that the case is a medically unambiguous one. In his discussion of treatment approaches to Patient C, Dr. Levy comments that "it is difficult to believe all the facts in this case. In particular, Patient C's various underlying disease states and abnormal laboratory values seem incompatible with a normal, alert mental status." In any case, Dr. Roy-Shapira is exactly right when he notes that Patient C's self-destructive behaviors ought not to determine whether he is admitted and treated. "To judge that the life of this patient is not worth living is making a quality-of-life decision. I do not think that physicians should be allowed to make quality-of-life decisions." Precisely. And that, I think, is why one cannot rightly base medical futility decisions on resultant quality of life.

In the United States, Dr. Chalfin would treat Patient B as long as some hope of benefit exists. He notes that in ICUs where a critical care physician is present, he or she can open lines of communication with the family and "work toward a humane and reasoned resolution that factors in the family's concerns and the patient's grave prognosis." This is of course consistent with the general legal and ethical consensus in the United States. In addition, he notes a point also made by Dr. Hoyt in his analysis of Patient A's case: ICUs work better when care is coordinated by intensivists rather than fragmented among many specialists.

Relative to Patient C, Dr. Chalfin notes "the disparities in American medicine . . . clearly the haves and have-nots often receive different care. Poor or absent indemnity coverage has an impact on patient health and access to medical care. In addition, hospitals that treat a large number of uninsured patients often face severe financial pressure and budgetary crises." This underlines one of the most obvious problems resulting from the United States' refusal to insure all its residents. Because Americans do not want to let people die from treatable illnesses (Americans claim that their medicine is the best in the world, after all), and because the country refuses to entertain universal health coverage, hospitals are forced to bear the burden. The result is that those hospitals that take seriously the ethical obligation to care for the poor and the uninsured are among the most likely to be forced to close. This has hit religion-affiliated hospitals especially hard. I do not mean to say here that America needs all the hospitals it has. Many cities are greatly overbedded. And many hospitals have failed at fiscal responsibility. But the present health care system in the United States is, I think, on a collision course with itself. The contradictory claims that people should get all the care they want and not pay for it simply cannot be sustained.

I will conclude with a few words about Dr. Crippen's commentary on Patient C's case. Because I am very typical of the ethicist he describes, I think I should respond as I would have done, had I been directly involved in this case. First, I have already spoken of the time issue and I admit it is indeed hard to determine it. Cases like this have made me think about this question of time more than I had before, and the result is what I have suggested earlier in this book.

Dr. Crippen suggests that an ethicist might feel in his "heart of hearts that the patient's desires should have been granted, on humanitarian grounds. It was physically possible to prop the patient up for a variable period longer. It should have been his right, living as he did in a society that spends huge amounts of money on other totally frivolous endeavors." I disagree. The present American health care system is an unethical mess. Dr. Crippen is quite right to say that treating Patient C is wrongheaded (again, assuming that the case is unambiguous, something questioned by Drs. Levy and Roy-Shapira). But the fault lies in the kind of system that American medicine has insisted on, where doctors and hospitals want to be free of governmental and societal restraint. That used to mean that they would insist on all sorts of silly treatment that patients and families tried to refuse—and get paid for them, by the way. In the 1970s, American courts finally began to recognize that patients and families had rights, too. They could make the value decisions. With the exceptions and restrictions I have noted, they could say yes or no to life-sustaining treatment. Now that hospitals and physicians do *not* get paid for overtreating patients, the worm has turned.

As I have said already, I wish there were some sort of societal agreement in the United States, explicit if at all possible, that would say to patients or families demanding treatment in cases like this one (again, assuming a lack of ambiguity in the case—Patient C really is in an inevitable and short-term death spiral) that there are simply no resources to pay for it. Justice demands a better use of these monies. These agreements, rejecting the kind of individualism that has served as the ethos for health care in America, are common throughout the world, as this book demonstrates so clearly. So "in my heart of hearts," I wanted then and want now for Patient C to accept his death, believe the doctors when they tell him no treatment can help, and ask for good palliation as he dies. But he did not want to do that—hence the conundrum. Dr. Crippen wants to avoid the problem by returning authority to physicians to decide about value-laden decisions. But that is what got society into this mess in the first place. I share his frustration. I do not accept his solution.

Summary

It seems, then, that neither for Patient A nor for Patient B can life-sustaining treatment be said to be medically futile. But as with Patient C, whose treatment might reasonably be considered medically futile, that does not mean it ought to be given. Different countries have differing social agreements, both explicit and implicit, that result in the limitation of treatment as part of a scheme for allocating limited resources to and within health care. Ethical analyses of these agreements would depend on an in-depth understanding of the many factors, economic and cultural, that go into their emergence. Even then there are no easy answers about where it is right to draw the lines. But as the varying actions and analyses of this book demonstrate, these hard issues must be faced.

References

[1]Ratiu P, Singer P: The ethics and economics of heroic surgery. Hastings Cent Rep 2001;31:47–8.

[2]*In re Helga Wanglie,* Fourth Judicial District (Dist Ct, Probate Ct Div 1991) PX-91-283. Minnesota, Hennepin County.

[3]National Conference of Catholic Bishops: Ethical and Religious Directives for Catholic Health Care Services. Washington, DC: USCCB Publishing, 2001.

Waiting for the Cavalry
The Role of the Courts in Recognizing Medical Futility

Jack K. Kilcullen, MD, JD, MPH

Profoundly ill patients continually confront the question of how hard to hold on. Often this falls to their families, who struggle to untangle their own feelings from those they believe their loved ones hold. The physician has a privileged role to play, serving as an advocate for life and a shepherd toward death. Every effort invested in this relationship over the years comes down to the days when the consent to treatment and the decision to forgo further care must be thoughtfully discussed so that a consensus can be reached.

Otherwise, courts are asked to step in. For hospitals and physicians, they seek judicial protection for the decisions to withhold or withdraw useless treatments, decisions grounded in the science and principles of the profession. For patients and their families wanting treatment to continue, they ask for help against overarching physician power. They want only to preserve the last precious moments of personal autonomy.

Courts have accomplished the task of protecting patients from treatment they do not want, in part because this involved the simpler task of patients' withdrawing from the relationship with the physician. With regard to patients seeking a level of care that doctors and hospitals believe falls far outside the standard, the few decisions the courts have made are inconsistent, involve applications of federal statutes in mechanical fashion, and fundamentally fail to address the implications for professional ethics and health care resource allocation. The lack of clarity has served only to further impair the medical profession in its already problematic mission of reaching a consensus of its own. As a result, intensive care unit (ICU) physicians faced daily with difficult triage decisions must remain very much alone.

The Easy Part: The Right to Refuse Treatment

The court in the landmark case *In re Quinlan,* the New Jersey Supreme Court, faced the case of a young woman whose medical condition and the dilemma it posed were described as follows:

A. . . . [Y]ou've got a set of possible lesions [in the brain] that prior to the era of advanced technology and advances in medicine were no problem inasmuch as the patient would expire. They could do nothing for themselves and even external care was limited. It was—I don't know how many years ago they couldn't keep a person alive with intravenous feedings because they couldn't give enough calories. Now they have these high caloric tube feedings that can keep people in excellent nutrition for years so what's happened is these things have occurred all along but the technology has now reached a point where you can in fact start to replace anything outside of the brain to maintain something that is irreversibly damaged.

Q. Doctor, can the art of medicine repair the cerebral damage that was sustained by Karen?

A. In my opinion, no. . . .

Q. Doctor, in your opinion is there any course of treatment that will lead to the improvement of Karen's condition?

A. No.[1]

The Supreme Court of Delaware wrote under similar facts in *Severns v Wilmington Medical Center, Inc.*:

Now, however, we are on the threshold of new terrain—the penumbra where death begins but life, in some form, continues. We have been led to it by the medical miracles which now compel us to distinguish between "death," as we have known it, and death in which the body lives in some fashion but the brain (or a significant part of it) does not.[2]

Whereas the state has the traditional interest in preserving life,[3] the individual has the fundamental freedom to refuse the medical treatment that life requires. This right stems from the common law of informed consent as well as from rights under the United States Constitution.[4] The Florida Supreme Court, in *Satz v Perlmutter*,[5] articulated this in recognizing the importance of honoring the privacy and dignity of both competent and incompetent persons. In the case of a paralyzed but competent patient with advanced amyotrophic lateral sclerosis, who sought removal of a respirator, the court embraced the lower court's reasoning:

It is all very convenient to insist on continuing Mr. Perlmutter's life so that there can be no question of foul play, no resulting civil liability and no possible trespass on medical ethics. However, it is quite another matter to do so at the patient's sole expense and against his competent will, thus inflicting never ending physical torture on his body until the inevitable, but artificially suspended, moment of death. Such a course of conduct invades the patient's constitutional right of privacy, removes his freedom of choice and invades his right to self-determine.[6]

The inability of a patient to express his or her wishes has been no bar to their being respected. The Massachusetts court, in *Brophy v New England Sinai Hospital, Inc.,*[7] had before it an application to end tube feedings for a man left in a persistent vegetative state from a subarachnoid hemorrhage. The case was brought by his wife and was opposed by his physicians. The court wrote:

> It is in recognition of these fundamental principles of individual autonomy that we . . . shift the emphasis away from a paternalistic view of what is "best" for a patient toward a reaffirmation that the basic question is what decision will comport with the will of the person involved, whether that person be competent or incompetent. As to the latter type of person, we concluded that the doctrine of substituted judgment, while not without its shortcomings, best serves to emphasize the importance of honoring the privacy and dignity of the individual. . . . To protect the incompetent person within its power, the State must recognize the dignity and worth of such a person and afford to that person the same panoply of rights and choices it recognizes in competent persons.[8]

As the court of Massachusetts noted, the interests of society over the fate of the gravely ill include the preservation of life, the protection of interests of innocent third parties, the prevention of suicide, and the maintenance of the ethical integrity of the medical profession. Specifically, the court observed that Mr. Brophy was not terminally ill or in danger of imminent death from any underlying physical illness. While acknowledging the trial judge's view that insertion of a gastrostomy tube (G-tube) is not a highly invasive or intrusive procedure and might not subject him to pain or suffering, the higher court faulted him for having "failed to consider that Brophy's judgment would be that being maintained by use of the G-tube is indeed intrusive. Additionally, in our view, the maintenance of Brophy . . . for a period of several years, is intrusive treatment as matter of law."[9]

Courts have therefore enforced the request of family members as guardians to withhold or withdraw medical and other invasive supportive care from patients who provided clear expression of their wishes. The United States Supreme Court established that the constitutional right of liberty and privacy would not prevent the state from requiring a heightened standard of evidence, that it be "clear and convincing."[10] Nor would a court require a hospital whose staff felt ethically compelled to provide continued care to withhold it; the family would be allowed instead to transfer the patient to a more obliging institution.[11] Furthermore, these cases arose in the setting of patients in a persistent vegetative state, a condition defined with clearly stated terms.[12]

Nevertheless, as the courts have recognized that the state's interest in preserving life pales before the protection of an individual's liberty, the power of the patient has grown dramatically. The patient, not the physician, decides that he or she is slowly dying, not simply still living. With this newly recognized control over the very terms of the discussion, patients and families have come to seek the opposite: that life be preserved.

Helga Wanglie and the Right to Require Treatment

In December 1989, Helga Wanglie, age 86, fractured her hip when she slipped on a rug in her Minneapolis, Minnesota, home. After the surgical repair performed at Hennepin County Medical Center (HCMC), she was discharged to a nursing home. Within a month, she was readmitted for respiratory failure and was placed on a ventilator. Mrs. Wanglie was conscious, aware of her surroundings, could acknowledge pain and suffering, and could recognize her family.

Over the next 5 months, repeated attempts to wean Mrs. Wanglie from the respirator were unsuccessful. In May 1990, she was transferred to a facility that specializes in the care of respirator-dependent patients. When further attempts were made to wean her, she experienced a cardiopulmonary arrest, was resuscitated, and was transferred first to another acute care hospital in St. Paul, Minnesota, and later back to HCMC. As a consequence of the arrest, she was considered to have extremely severe and irreversible brain damage. Despite this, she continued on a ventilator, receiving antibiotics for recurrent pneumonia, artificial feeding, and treatment for electrolyte and fluid imbalances. Her readmission diagnosis of persistent vegetative state secondary to severe hypoxic-ischemic encephalopathy was confirmed repeatedly over the next several months by the hospital neurology service. Hospital pulmonologists confirmed as well that she had become permanently ventilator-dependent because of chronic lung disease.

Because of her age and her prolonged hospital stay at HCMC, marked by multiple complications and the failure to wean her from the ventilator, the medical staff caring for Mrs. Wanglie viewed her prognosis as poor. Several family conferences were held in November and December. The family was told that the attending physicians caring for Mrs. Wanglie had concluded that continued use of the respirator could not serve the patient's interests. A conference was held with hospital staff, the Wanglie family, and Dr. Steven Miles, a representative of the hospital ethics committee and the petitioner in this case. After this conference, Oliver Wanglie wrote in a letter, "My wife always stated to me that if anything happened to her so that she could not take care of herself, she did not want anything done to shorten or prematurely take her life."

In a letter to Mr. Wanglie, the hospital's medical director responded:

> All medical consultants agree with [the attending physician's] conclusion that continued use of mechanical ventilation and other forms of life-sustaining treatment are no longer serving the patient's personal medical interest. We do not believe that the hospital is obliged to provide inappropriate medical treatment that cannot advance a patient's personal interest. We would continue life-sustaining treatment on the order of a court mandating such treatment. In view of the extraordinary nature of your request [to continue treatment], we ask that you file petition to obtain such an order by December 14.[13]

When it appeared that the family was not going to initiate proceedings, the hospital filed its own petition with the Fourth Judicial District Court, Hennepin County, in February 1991, seeking an independent guardian. At that point, Mr. Wanglie filed for conservatorship, and it was this application that the court approved.[14] The judge ruled that the husband was "in the best position to investigate and act upon Helga Wanglie's conscientious, religious, and moral beliefs." Three days after the decision, Mrs. Wanglie died from sepsis. Her care was paid for by a private insurer, a health maintenance organization, which agreed to do so notwithstanding the opinion of the doctors and the hospital. The total cost was estimated at $700,000.[15]

The case spawned articles and editorials in the bioethics and medical literature, not to mention the popular press.[16] However, the legal issue was a routine probate concern about the suitability of a spouse's serving as guardian, which in other circumstances would have occurred without notice. Given the forum, the physicians' hope for relief was ill placed. Whereas they hoped for a discussion of the ethical challenges they sincerely faced, it was clear before the court that Mr. Wanglie was his wife's best advocate and on this fact alone, his application was properly granted. In less than 2 years, the debate would resume, only this time with the physicians even more on the defensive. A federal law to help the indigent would become a powerful means to challenge a broad range of physician conduct on behalf of anyone seeking hospital care.

Not Exactly What They Had in Mind:
Congress, The Right to Emergency Treatment,
and the Case of Baby K

In October 1992, a woman in Fairfax, Virginia, gave birth by cesarean section to a child known for months to be profoundly impaired. Lacking a cerebral cortex and part of the skull and scalp, this anencephalic child went immediately into respiratory distress on birth and was intubated and put on a mechanical ventilator. The doctors had no illusion about the child's prognosis; indeed, much earlier they had included terminating the pregnancy among the options presented to the mother. They saw this aggressive intervention as only a temporizing gesture to help the mother come to terms with this fatal diagnosis. As the Society of Critical Care Medicine would later argue in their friend-of-the-court brief, anencephalic infants are "so impaired that treatment will serve only to maintain biologic functions."[17] Although the physicians recommended hydration and warmth, the mother insisted that the infant receive aggressive intervention. After 6 weeks, Baby K, as she would come to be known, was successfully weaned and was transferred to a nursing home.

Baby K returned to the hospital in January 1993 after experiencing bradypnea and apnea requiring ventilatory support. Hospital officials sought once more to persuade the mother to discontinue ventilator treatment, and she again refused. After Baby K could breathe on her own, she was transferred back to the nursing home in February 1993, but within weeks, she was back in the hospital requiring reintubation. A tracheostomy was performed in March 1993, and the patient was returned to the nursing home.

The hospital sought judicial review to relieve it of the burden of forestalling what it considered an inevitable demise. It brought its action in federal court under a provision of the very law that was its biggest obstacle: the federal Emergency Treatment and Active Labor Act (EMTALA).[18] Seven years earlier, in 1986, Congress had taken action against the nationwide practice of patient dumping, where individuals with emergency conditions were barred from private emergency departments (EDs) because they lacked evidence of health insurance.[19] In fact, less than half the states posed any legal requirements on hospitals to provide emergency care, with a majority of these lacking any meaningful enforcement mechanism.[20] Traditional common-law imposed no burden on hospitals whatsoever.[21]

Now, any hospital caring for patients receiving federal funds, only in the form of reimbursement for care administered to Medicare or Medicaid patients, had two responsibilities. It must screen anyone seeking treatment for an emergency condition, and it must stabilize that condition before arranging safe transfer to a facility covered by that patient's insurance or where more sophisticated care may be received.

> In the case of a hospital that has a hospital emergency department, if any individual (whether or not eligible for benefits under this subchapter) comes to the emergency department and a request is made on the individual's behalf for examination or treatment for a medical condition, the hospital must provide for an appropriate medical screening examination within the capability of the hospital's emergency department, including ancillary services routinely available to the emergency department, to determine whether or not an emergency medical condition (within the meaning of subsection (e)(1) of this section) exists. . . .[22]
>
> . . . An emergency condition is defined broadly to include: a medical condition manifesting itself by acute symptoms of sufficient severity (including severe pain) such that the absence of immediate medical attention could reasonably be expected to result in—
>> (i) placing the health of the individual . . . in serious jeopardy,
>> (ii) serious impairment to bodily functions, or
>> (iii) serious dysfunction of any bodily organ or part.[23]

If the hospital discovered an emergency condition, it must stabilize the patient or transfer the patient to a facility with the necessary resources, assuming the benefits of the transfer were outweighed by the risks:

> [T]he hospital must provide either—
>> (A) within the staff and facilities available at the hospital, for such further medical examination and such treatment as may be required to stabilize the medical condition, or
>> (B) for the transfer of the individual to another medical facility in accordance with subsection (c) of this section.[24]

The treatment required "to stabilize" a patient is that treatment "necessary to assure, within reasonable medical probability, that no material deterioration of the condition is likely to result from or occur . . ."[25]

The hospital argued that Baby K's diagnosis was anencephaly and that this condition, not the immediate respiratory distress, should be at the heart of the plan of care. Whereas the respiratory distress might in fact be treatable, the anencephaly was not. On that basis, aggressive treatment was not indicated. The hospital argued that the federal statute should not be construed as covering care that the hospital considered to be not only futile but inhumane.

The trial court rejected the argument:

> The plain language of the statute requires stabilization of an emergency medical condition. The statute does not admit of any "futility" or "inhumanity" exceptions. Any argument to the contrary should be directed to the U.S. Congress, not to the Federal Judiciary.[26]

The court went further:

> Even if EMTALA contained the exceptions advanced by the Hospital, these exceptions would not apply here. The use of a mechanical ventilator to assist breathing is not "futile" or "inhumane" in relieving the acute symptoms of respiratory difficulty which is the emergency medical condition that must be treated under EMTALA. To hold otherwise would allow hospitals to deny emergency treatment to numerous classes of patients, such as accident victims who have terminal cancer or AIDS [acquired immunodeficiency syndrome], on the grounds that they eventually will die anyway from those diseases and that emergency care for them would therefore be "futile."[27]

In short order, the court held that EMTALA directed the hospital to respond to any immediate emergency requiring stabilizing treatment.

Building on its description of Baby K as a member of a definable class of disabled persons, the court turned to antidiscrimination statutes aimed at protecting individuals with disabilities. Starting with the Rehabilitation Act of 1973,[28] which bars recipients of federal funds from discrimination, the court wrote:

> When the Rehabilitation Act was passed in 1973, Congress intended that discrimination on the basis of a handicap be treated in the same manner that Title VI of the Civil Rights Act treats racial

discrimination. . . . This analogy to race dispels any ambiguity about the extent to which Baby K has statutory rights not to be discriminated against on the basis of her handicap. *It also shatters the Hospital's contention that ventilator treatment should be withheld because Baby K's recurring breathing troubles are intrinsically related to her handicap.* No such distinction would be permissible within the context of racial discrimination. In addition, the Hospital was able to perform a tracheotomy on Baby K. This surgery was far more complicated than linking her to a ventilator to allow her to breathe. . . . Just as an AIDS patient seeking ear surgery is "otherwise qualified" to receive treatment despite poor long term prospects of living, Baby K is "otherwise qualified" to receive ventilator treatment despite similarly dismal health prospects. . . . Thus, the Hospital's desire to withhold ventilator treatment from Baby K over her mother's objections would violate the Rehabilitation Act.[29] (emphasis added)

Characterizing hospital care as a "public accommodation," the court wielded section 302(a) of the Americans With Disabilities Act (ADA)[30] in similar fashion. This provision states: "No individual shall be discriminated against on the basis of disability in the full and equal enjoyment of . . . public accommodations." The court stated:

The Hospital asks this court for authorization to deny the benefits of ventilator services to Baby K by reason of her anencephaly. The Hospital's claim is that it is "futile" to keep alive an anencephalic baby, even though the mother has requested such treatment. But the plain language of the ADA does not permit the denial of ventilator services that would keep alive an anencephalic baby when those life-saving services would otherwise be provided to a baby without disabilities at the parent's request. The Hospital's reasoning would lead to the denial of medical services to anencephalic babies as a class of disabled individuals. Such discrimination against a vulnerable population class is exactly what the American with Disabilities Act was enacted to prohibit.[31]

Essential to its arguments was its continued separation of Baby K's anencephaly from her repeated respiratory crises, when this very repetition intrinsic to her congenital defects was what prompted the hospital to go to court. In contrast, the United States Supreme Court, in *Bowen v American Hospital Association,* referred to federal guidelines under the Rehabilitation Act regarding the nature of anencephaly as precisely that special handicap that can justify the withholding of treatment:

Section 504 does not require treatment of anencephaly because it would "do no more than temporarily prolong the act of dying"); para. (a)(iv) (same with severely premature and low birth weight infants). In general, the guidelines seem to make a hospital's liability under § 504 dependent on proof that (1) it refused to provide requested treatment or nourishment solely on the basis of an infant's handicapping condition, and (2) the treatment or nourishment *would have been medically beneficial.*[32] (emphasis added)

However, this dictum was not considered by the trial court.

The Court of Appeals for the Fourth Circuit simplified the reasoning without changing the result. Resting exclusively on EMTALA, the court rejected each of the hospital's arguments. First, it considered the hospital's position that in prohibiting disparate emergency medical treatment, Congress did not intend to require physicians to provide treatment outside the prevailing standard of medical care, with the premise that anencephaly was the primary diagnosis.

Relying on [previous] decisions of this court, the Hospital contends that it is only required to provide Baby K with the same treatment that it would provide other anencephalic infants—supportive care in the form of warmth, nutrition, and hydration. . . . Advancing the proposition that anencephaly, as opposed to respiratory distress, is the emergency medical condition at issue, the Hospital concludes that it is only required to provide uniform treatment to all anencephalic infants. We disagree. . . .

. . . It is bradypnea or apnea, not anencephaly, that is the emergency medical condition that brings Baby K to the Hospital for treatment. Uniform treatment of emergency medical conditions would require the Hospital to provide Baby K with the same treatment that the Hospital provides all other patients experiencing bradypnea or apnea. The Hospital does not allege that it would refuse to provide respiratory support to infants experiencing bradypnea or apnea who do not have anencephaly. Indeed, a refusal to provide such treatment would likely be considered as providing no emergency medical treatment. . . .

. . . the plain language of EMTALA requires stabilizing treatment for any individual who comes to a participating hospital, is diagnosed as having an emergency medical condition, and cannot be transferred. . . . The Hospital has been unable to identify, nor has our research revealed, any statutory language or legislative history evincing a Congressional intent to create an exception to the duty to provide stabilizing treatment when the required treatment would exceed the prevailing standard of medical care. *We recognize the dilemma facing physicians who are requested to provide treatment they consider morally and ethically inappropriate, but we cannot ignore the plain language of the statute because to do so would transcend our judicial function.* . . . The appropriate branch to redress the policy concerns of the Hospital is Congress.[33] (emphasis added)

Second, the court considered the hospital's argument that EMTALA was limited by Virginia law, which required doctors to adhere to professional standards and thus withhold inappropriate treatment. This, too, was disposed of by the court. Citing the supremacy of federal law, the court wrote:

The duty to provide stabilizing treatment set forth in EMTALA applies not only to participating hospitals but also to treating physicians in participating hospitals. EMTALA does not provide an exception for stabilizing treatment physicians may deem medically or ethically inappropriate. Consequently, to the extent [Va. Code Ann] § 54.1–2990 exempts physicians from providing care they consider medically or ethically inappropriate, it directly conflicts with the provisions of EMTALA that require stabilizing treatment to be provided.[34]

The child continued to live in a nursing home, with the hospital required to provide emergency care. By the time she reached age 2, the bills had exceeded $400,000, covered by the mother's health insurance.[35] Six months later, Baby K died from a cardiac arrest.[36]

The Fourth Circuit rode its plain-language view of EMTALA far beyond the constraints of the statute's legislative purpose of preventing discrimination against the indigent, joined in the journey by the majority of other circuits under a panoply of circumstances. For instance, in *Gatewood v Washington Healthcare Corporation*,[37] an action claiming inadequate medical screening was brought by the surviving wife of a man who died from a heart attack after being sent home from the ED with a diagnosis of musculoskeletal pain. The trial court had dismissed the action in part on the grounds that the patient was insured and thus outside the intended scope of EMTALA. Though affirming dismissal by the trial court, the Court of Appeals for the First Circuit specifically rejected the trials court's rationale:

We find that the District Court erred in relying on Mr. Gatewood's insured status for its holding. Though the Emergency Act's legislative history reflects an unmistakable concern with the treatment of uninsured patients, the Act itself draws no distinction between persons with and without insurance. Rather, the Act's plain language unambiguously extends its protections to "*any* individual" who seeks emergency room assistance.[38]

The United States Supreme Court recently endorsed this plain-text view in reversing the Sixth Circuit decision in *Roberts v Galen*[39] by striking down the lower court's requirement that there be shown an "improper motive" behind a hospital's failure to make efforts to stabilize the patient.

In the wake of *In re Baby K* and other decisions, courts continue to rein in the cases taking advantage of the expansive scope the courts created for EMTALA. In particular, they struggle to prevent its becoming a federal malpractice law, which Congress had no intention of seeing happen.[40] Within 2 years, the Fourth Circuit was faced with the question of how long after admission EMTALA applied. In *Bryan v Rectors and Visitors of the Univ. of Va.,*[41] the patient, Shirley Robertson, was transferred from one hospital to the University of Virginia Medical Center in respiratory distress. Over the next 12 days, aggressive treatment ensued consistent with the family's wishes that all necessary measures be taken to keep her alive, with "trust in God's wisdom." Without the family's consent, the hospital physicians ultimately entered a do-not-resuscitate order, and within days the patient died.

Factually, the issue before the court was the duration of the stabilizing requirement of EMTALA. In this case, the court noted:

> As is admitted in the complaint, and so necessarily conceded by Bryan in her brief and oral argument, stabilizing treatment was provided by the hospital from Robertson's arrival on February 5 until February 17. But, the claim is that the hospital's abandonment of such treatment as of its entering the anti-resuscitation order on February 17 and its failure to offer stabilizing treatment in response to Robertson's heart attack eight days later constituted an EMTALA violation.[42]

In stark contrast to its disregard of the legislative history in *In re Baby K,* the court wrote that EMTALA's

> core purpose is to get patients into the system who might otherwise go untreated and be left without a remedy because traditional medical malpractice law affords no claim for failure to treat.[43]

The plaintiff argued that the court was saying instead that

> without regard to professional standards of care or the standards embodied in the state law of medical malpractice, the hospital would have to provide treatment indefinitely—perhaps for years—according to a novel, federal standard of care derived from the statutory stabilization requirement. We do not find this reading of the statute plausible.[44]

The Ninth Circuit reached a similar conclusion in *James v Sunrise Hospital*.[45] In that case, a woman was admitted to Sunrise Hospital with acute renal failure. In preparation for hemodialysis, the hospital inserted a synthetic graft into her arm. The next day, she complained of pain and numbness in that forearm, wrist, and hand. Two days later, the woman's pain and numbness had spread. Hospital personnel examined her and found that her hand was cool and beginning to turn blue. These complaints continued, and 5 days later, hospital personnel noted that the pulse in the arm was also weak. Nevertheless, she was discharged without any evaluation of the condition of her veins. This condition was not stabilized before her discharge and subsequently led to amputation of her hand.

Although other courts have held that under EMTALA, a hospital must actually be aware of a patient's emergency condition before it can be held liable for failing to stabilize it,[46] the court in this case was not willing to do so.[47] Instead, it focused on language under subsection (c) concerning transfer of patients that makes reference to "emergency department" personnel to suggest that these patients being transferred were leaving the ED and had not spent days on the floor:

> Thus we read the transfer restrictions of 42 U.S.C. § 1395dd(c) to apply only when an individual "comes to the emergency room," and after "an appropriate medical screening examination," "the hospital determines that the individual has an emergency medical condition."[48]

Not so to the Sixth Circuit. In *Thornton v Southwest Detroit Hospital,* an action was brought on behalf of a woman who had a stroke and was admitted to the ICU, where she spent 10 days, followed by 11 days on a regular ward. Because she did not have the insurance to pay for placement in a specialized rehabilitation facility, she was discharged to her sister's, where her condition deteriorated. She was then admitted to another facility. The suit alleged that she was not sufficiently stabilized before her discharge.

The legal issue for the court concerned the relationship between the two duties EMTALA places on hospitals—to screen and to stabilize. Section 42 U.S.C. §1395dd(a) states that

> if any individual . . . comes *to the emergency department* and a request is made on the individual's behalf for examination or treatment for a medical condition, *the hospital must provide for an appropriate medical screening examination* within the capability of the hospital's emergency department. (emphasis added)

In broader terms, 42 U.S.C. §1395dd(b)(1) states that

> if they discovered an emergency condition, they must stabilize the patient or transfer the patient to a facility with the necessary resources, assuming the benefits of the transfer were outweighed by the risks.

Had EMTALA been targeted by the courts as it had been by Congress toward people without insurance who were being denied emergency treatment, the scope of treatment would be confined to the time of the patient's arrival and not throughout his or her stay as the Fourth Circuit held. The Sixth Circuit itself quoted reports from the House Judiciary Committee as well as its Ways and Means Committee about the lack of needed ED care for the indigent. Yet it nevertheless believed that

> [a] fairer reading is that Congress sought to insure that patients with medical emergencies would receive emergency care. Although emergency care often occurs, and almost invariably begins, in an emergency room, emergency care does not always stop when a patient is wheeled from the emergency room into the main hospital. Hospitals may not circumvent the requirements of the Act merely by admitting an emergency room patient to the hospital, then immediately discharging that patient. Emergency care must be given until the patient's emergency medical condition is stabilized.[49]

According to its view of the facts, no emergency existed at the time of discharge, and so the hospital was not at fault. But its position was clear: EMTALA has jurisdiction over any claim of a patient not adequately stabilized, regardless of how much time has elapsed since his or her admission. Other courts have read the two sections disjunctively,[50] though in *Smith v Richmond Mem'l Hosp.*[51] and *Lopez-Soto v Hawayek*,[52] the patient was an infant whose emergency condition arose during delivery.

The United States Supreme Court, in *Roberts v Galen,* gave implied legitimacy to EMTALA's reach long into a person's hospital stay. In May 1992, a woman suffered severe injuries after being hit by a truck. After 6 weeks of rigorous care at a Humana hospital in Louisville, Kentucky, she remained subject to fevers and changes in blood pressure. Humana nevertheless succeeded in arranging her transfer to an extended health care facility nearby. Yet shortly after the transfer, her condition once again began to deteriorate. The lower court had granted summary judgment for the hospital on the grounds that an improper motive was required and not shown. The Court rejected that requirement and sent the case back for further proceedings.[53] However, the fact that the case was allowed to continue suggests that 6 weeks is no outright bar to an action under EMTALA.

Indeed, that was the position one government lawyer argued before the Court in *Roberts.* Enforcement of EMTALA is shared by the Centers for Medicare & Medicaid Services (formerly the Health Care Financing Administration [HCFA]) of the Department of Health and Human Services (HHS) and HHS' Office of Inspector General (OIG). The fact that the Supreme Court chose a case to discuss EMTALA involving a patient whose emergency occurred weeks after her arrival at the ED carries the implicit assumption that EMTALA reaches deep into the inpatient world. A top official in the OIG was quoted as saying, "The IG's [Inspector General's] view is that the EMTALA statute covers patients who are in a hospital and are unstable." The OIG and the Centers for Medicare & Medicaid Services have yet to fulfill their announced intention of providing joint guidance on EMTALA's power and scope. In a conference call with representatives of the American Hospital Association, Gloria Frank, then HCFA's lead enforcement official on EMTALA, was asked:

> Q4: Has HCFA formally adopted a position concerning whether EMTALA applies to inpatient admissions?
> Answer: No, not yet. HCFA and OIG are currently formulating their national, formal position on this issue. Note: Pending such a national formal position, providers should contact their regional office to ascertain their regional offices' position on this issue. Some regional offices have asserted that EMTALA applies to a limited class of inpatients. To my knowledge, some of the regions occasionally take a case where the patient was an inpatient for a short period of time and was never stabilized. Overall, providers may want to maintain the status quo until HCFA sets forth a national, formal position on this issue.[54]

Getting Back to Basics:
The Standard of Care and the Refusal to Treat

Ultimately, the determination that care is medically futile is, from a court's point of view, the responsibility of the medical profession. Indeed, the judge relies on physicians acting as expert witnesses to guide him or her in determining whether another physician's conduct was negligent. The issue was framed with remarkable clarity in *Causey v St. Francis Med. Ctr.*[55] In that case, a physician and hospital, believing it medically appropriate to do so, withdrew life-sustaining care from a 31-year-old, quadriplegic, comatose patient with end-stage renal failure, over the strongly expressed objections of the patient's family. A former employee of the defendant hospital, Sonya Causey, experienced complications during childbirth and was left essentially quadriplegic. She was transferred to the Oak Wood Nursing Home in Mer Rouge, Louisiana. Thereafter, she underwent dialysis three times a week at St. Francis Medical Center (SFMC) in Pittsburgh, Pennsylvania. A permanent tracheal tube was placed to assist her in breathing. At the time of this incident, she had end-stage renal disease, diabetes mellitus, hypertension, and quadriplegia. In October 1996, she developed respiratory distress and was taken by ambulance to Morehouse General Hospital. She experienced cardiopulmonary arrest and was transferred to SFMC in a comatose condition. She remained at SFMC until her death on November 22, 1996. At that time she was diagnosed with stage IV coma, secondary to at least three or four cardiopulmonary arrests.

Although the physician, Dr. Herschel Harter, agreed at the time of the patient's hospitalization at SFMC that with dialysis and a ventilator Mrs. Causey could live for another 2 years, he believed that she would have only a slight (1%–5%) chance of regaining consciousness. Because Mrs. Causey's family demanded aggressive life-sustaining care, Dr. Harter sought (unsuccessfully) to transfer her to another medical facility willing to provide this care. Dr. Harter enlisted support from SFMC's Morals and Ethics Board. The board agreed with Dr. Harter that dialysis and life-support procedures should be stopped and that a "no-code" status (do-not-resuscitate orders) should be entered. The feeding tube was withdrawn, and use of other similar devices ceased. The day the ventilator was removed, Mrs. Causey died from respiratory and cardiac failure.[56]

The family brought the action before a state trial court in Louisiana and characterized it as an intentional battery-based tort, claiming a lack of consent to the defendants' treatment decision. But the trial court found that the defendants "acted in accordance with professional opinions and professional judgment" and thus this action was covered by Louisiana's Medical

Malpractice Act,[57] which required that it first be presented to a medical review panel. Accordingly, the trial court dismissed the action as premature.[58]

The appellate court faced the question of futility squarely. After discussing the line of cases articulating a patient's right to refuse treatment, the court wrote:

> Now the roles are reversed. Patients or, if incompetent, their surrogate decision-makers, are demanding life-sustaining treatment regardless of its perceived futility, while physicians are objecting to being compelled to prolong life with procedures they consider futile. The right or autonomy of the patient to refuse treatment is simply a severing of the relationship with the physician. In this case, however, the patient (through her surrogate) is not severing a relationship, but demanding treatment the physician believes is "inappropriate."[59]

The court recognized that "[f]utility is a subjective and nebulous concept." It relegated EMTALA and the ADA to a footnote as distractions from the moral complexities at hand.[60] It went on:

> Placement of statistical cut-off points for futile treatment involves subjective value judgments. The difference in opinion as to whether a 2% or 9% probability of success is the critical point for determining futility can be explained in terms of personal values, not in terms of medical science. When the medical professional and the patient, through a surrogate, disagree on the worth of pursuing life, this is a conflict over values, i.e., whether extra days obtained through medical intervention are worth the burden and costs. . . .[61]
>
> . . . Physicians are professionals and occupy a special place in our community. They are licensed by society to perform this special role. No one else is permitted to use life-prolonging technology, which is considered by many as "fundamental" health care. The physician has an obligation to present all medically acceptable treatment options for the patient or her surrogate to consider and either choose or reject; however, this does not compel a physician to provide interventions that in his view would be harmful, without effect or "medically inappropriate."[62]
>
> . . . A finding that treatment is "medically inappropriate" by a consensus of physicians practicing in that specialty translates into a standard of care. Thus, in this case, whether Dr. Harter and SFMC met the standard of care concerning the withdrawal of dialysis, life-support procedures and the entering of a "no code" status must be determined.[63]

As well it should be. Yet the debate over "medical futility" has been raging
and rumbling for years among members of the medical community, pitting
the authority of physicians against the autonomy of patients.[64] Thus, as a
definable standard, there are those, such as Dr. James F. Drane and Dr. John
L. Coulehan, who maintain that

> [a] patient's right to choose or refuse treatment is limited by the
> physician's right (and duty) to practice medicine responsibly. . . .
> Physicians . . . have a right to refuse to provide futile treatments
> (i.e., interventions that might be physiologically effective in some
> sense but cannot benefit a patient). Patients themselves have a right
> to provide input into what would constitute a "benefit" for them, but
> physicians should be able to decide when a particular treatment is
> futile based on their knowledge of the treatment's effects and its
> likely impact on a patient's quality of life.[65]

Others, such as Dr. Robert M. Veatch and Carol Mason Spicer, argue:

> Under certain circumstances patients should have the right to
> receive life-prolonging care from their clinicians . . . even if it
> violates their consciences to provide it. Society is not in a position
> to override a competent patient who prefers to live even if life
> prolongation is burdensome. For incompetent patients, if a clinician
> believes a treatment is actually hurting a patient significantly, he or
> she may appeal to a court to have it stopped. . . . A society that
> forces people to die against their will produces more offense than
> one that forces healthcare providers to provide services that violate
> their consciences.[66]

Courts are already challenged to decide the professional standard of
care in a routine malpractice case when the physician witnesses called as
experts sharply disagree over how a particular patient should have been
treated. The difficulty is compounded when the terms of the debate the
physicians use are grounded in personal values, rather than medical science.

To that end, Lawrence J. Schneiderman and other advocates of
physicians' terminating treatment deemed futile have labored to incorporate
their views into formal policies of various health care institutions.[67] For the
ICU physician, there are as well the standards the Society of Critical Care
Medicine provides for the allocation of scarce ICU resources[68]:

> Patients with little or no anticipated benefit from further ICU
> treatment may be discharged or transferred from the ICU. Patients

with terminal, irreversible illness who face imminent death should be excluded from the ICU. Very elderly individuals who are failing to thrive due to irreversible, chronic illness should not be encouraged to use intensive care. The decision to exclude or discharge a patient from the ICU may appropriately be made despite the anticipation of an untoward outcome.[69]

The difficulty associated with implementing decisions to terminate care is that the "untoward outcome" doctors anticipate may be a legal one. As Dr. Steve Heilig of the San Francisco Medical Society noted:

Contrary to assertions that there has been a decline in the futility movement and that futile treatment cannot be defined, many hospitals and other health care organizations have developed policies and procedures covering this area, and more will probably do so. . . . Such policies can include a careful and inclusive review of any putative case of nonbeneficial treatment, which would include talking to patients and their families about the treatment . . . and the use of second opinions, consultation with specialists, and review by an institutional ethics committee. In other words, the process is about as inclusive as is practicable. . . . During the lengthy process of developing such broad-based guidelines in northern California, there was a strong consensus that such policies were needed but that fears about liability precluded their implementation.[70]

And so, while physicians may wait for outside help, they do so with the ironic fear of intervention from the very authority whose decisions turn on guidance physicians themselves must provide. Absent that guidance, courts will be encouraged to fill the gap with federal laws never drafted to decide the question at hand.

All Patients Are Autonomous, but Some Are More Autonomous Than Others.

The "problem that won't go away" is that whereas courts grant patients equal autonomy, society has made little attempt to pay for it.[71] More than 40 million Americans without health insurance may have EMTALA to get them into the ED but not into a private physician's office. Baby K and Helga Wanglie had insurance providers willing to underwrite their care. What does a hospital do when a patient's family insists on aggressive treatment they have no means to pay for? Under EMTALA, they may attempt to transfer the patient only if there is an accepting institution.[72] But without private or

Medicare coverage or sufficient poverty to qualify for Medicaid, realistically there is nowhere else that patient can go.

Health care centers serving poor and uninsured individuals are struggling, even as they are lauded for their success at operating efficiently.[73] While investor-owned hospitals thrive, nonprofit and municipal facilities are closing.[74] Physician advocates for patient autonomy see the difficulty. As Dr. Veatch wrote:

> We have acknowledged the legitimacy and necessity of rationing healthcare, provided it is done equitably and with full public participation in decisions. But historically the clinician's job has been to help patients, not to act as society's cost-containment agent. This gatekeeping role must be someone else's task. Just like a defense attorney's role in the legal system is to advocate for a client, even an unworthy client, a clinician's job in the medical system is to advocate for his or her patient.
>
> We agree that care without effect should not be funded on scientific grounds. A clinician should not be permitted to authorize treatments that he or she is convinced will not produce the effect a patient or surrogate seeks. In fact, insurers who receive requests for reimbursement for such care ought not to pay for it. However, for care that affects the dying trajectory but seems to most of us to offer no benefit, the proper course is for society—not clinicians—to cut patients off. Subscribers to insurance should have a strong interest in limiting care that offers little or no benefit and should agree to exclude such coverage from their plans.

Where is the equity among patients when one has a carrier as generous as the Wanglies' and his or her neighbor does not? In fact, many with health insurance lack significant rights to sue their health maintenance organizations, who are protected by federal law from state law liability. This protection at the expense of the patient is one of the inducements established by Congress to encourage private health insurance to make up for the lack of universal coverage.[75] When a patient learns that he or she will not be reimbursed for care that has been deemed medically unnecessary, ironically that patient may have more rights to sue the hospital to continue care than he or she does to compel the insurer to pay for it.

For those without insurance, the costs of care not compensated for may be more dramatically felt when it means that public institutions must cut programs elsewhere to pay for care that a court may deem to be within a patient's rights. For example, the cost of Helga Wanglie's care exceeded the cost to New York City's public hospital system to run 17 school-based clinics for 6 months, clinics that the city may be compelled to close for lack of funds.[76] Thus, for patients relying on hospitals serving the underserved—hospitals whose resources are already stretched—the rights of a Helga Wanglie or a Baby K may exhaust the chance of many others who follow to claim rights to care far more modest, such as a checkup or a prescription.

Conclusion: Tickets to the Lifeboat

This discussion of finance serves to introduce scarcity to the futility debate. And where even the most deluxe insurance package is helpless is in creating an ICU bed when all are already taken. An ICU is a finite resource for the community it serves, however unlimited it may be theoretically in the future. Patients A, B, and C represent the spectrum of medical and ethical challenges daily facing ICU physicians who must allocate scarce beds. Moreover, these physicians must often choose among such patients, at least hypothetically, knowing that given the volume in their hospitals, Patient C may be in the ED but Patient A could arrive within days or hours. While the laws of society strive toward equality, the laws of nature remain capriciously unfair.

Working at the law's frontier, the ICU physician strives to give a scarce resource to the most deserving patient. Without a cavalry to prevent them from a desperate Patient C or the family of Patient B, physicians must save a bed for Patient A, even when he is still only lying on a stretcher in another hospital awaiting the disaster that will send him to the ICU. This duty, along with all the rest, is just part of the intensivist's job.

Futile treatment—that is, ICU treatment given to those who will not benefit from it—is not merely a luxury. It is the proximate reason for another's demise when it means that a desperately needed bed is still unavailable. Therefore, physicians at the local level, to whom courts turn when judging the behavior of physicians, must speak with a clearer voice about the purpose of the ICU: to restore a measure of a person's ability to function in his or her world. For the debilitated patient facing yet another admission, palliative care, not aggressive intervention, should be the professional standard of care to which physicians adhere. Patients already in the ICU who show no further progress may be discharged to a regular medical floor to make room for other patients, even if transfer may hasten their deaths. Given the paucity of judicial precedent, physicians and their lawyers must organize to articulate these principles so that there is no question for a court or a jury about what the standard of care should be. That standard should mean that those allowed in the lifeboat are those with the best chance of surviving the long trip home.

Notes

[1]*In re Quinlan,* 70 NJ 10, 20 (NJ 1976).

[2]421 A2d 1334, 1344 (Del 1980).

[3]*Brophy v New England Sinai Hospital, Inc.,* 398 Mass 417, 432 (Mass 1986).

[4]Laurence H. Tribe, *American Constitutional Law.* 2nd ed. Mineola, NY: Foundation Press, 1988, p. 1365.

[5]379 So2d 359 (Fla 1980).

[6]Id. at 164.

[7]398 Mass 417 (Mass 1986).

[8]*Brophy,* supra, at 430–1, quoting from its earlier decision in *Superintendent of Belchertown State School v Saikewicz,* 373 Mass 728, 740–1 (1977).

[9]*Brophy,* supra, at 434–5.

[10]*Cruzan v Missouri Department of Health,* 497 US 261 (1990).

[11]See, for example, *Brophy,* supra, at 442.

[12]*Brophy,* supra, at 421, n.4.

[13]Ronald E. Cranford, Department of Neurology, Hennepin County Medical Center, Minneapolis, Minnesota. Available at: http://www.missouri.edu/~philwb/anglie.html. Accessed November 9, 2001.

[14]*In re Helga Wanglie,* Fourth Judicial District (Dist Ct, Probate Ct Div 1991) PX-91-283. Minnesota, Hennepin County.

[15]Steven H. Miles, "Interpersonal Issues in the Wanglie Case," *Kennedy Institute of Ethics Journal* 2:61, 65, 1992.

[16]See, for example, Marcia Angell, "After Quinlan: The Dilemma of the Persistent Vegetative State," *New England Journal of Medicine* 330:1524–5, 1994; Tom L. Beauchamp and Robert M. Veatch, *Ethical Issues in Death and Dying.* 2nd ed. New York: Prentice Hall, 1995 (see notes xv–xvi).

[17]Brief of the Society of Critical Care Medicine as Amicus Curiae at 10–11, n.22, *In re Baby K,* 16 F3d 590, *cert denied,* 115 SCt 91 (1994).

[18]42 USC §1395dd (2001).

[19]Lynn Healey Scaduto, "The Emergency Medical Treatment and Active Labor Act Gone Astray: A Proposal to Reclaim EMTALA for Its Intended Beneficiaries," *UCLA Law Review* 46:943–82, 1999.

[20]Judith L. Dobbertin, "Eliminating Patient Dumping: A Proposal for Model Legislation," *Valparaiso University Law Review* 28:291, 323–31, 1993.

[21]Scaduto, op. cit. at n.2.

[22]42 USC §1395dd (a).

[23]42 USC §1395dd(e)(1)(A).

[24]42 USC §1395dd(b)(1).

[25]42 USC §1395dd(e)(3)(A).

[26]In The Matter of Baby K 832 F Supp 1022, 1027 (EDVa 1993).

[27]Id. at 1029.

[28]29 USC 794 et seq.

[29]Id. at 1028.

[30]42 USC §12101 et seq.

[31]Id. at 1029.

[32]*Bowen v American Hospital Association,* 476 US 610, 614 n.4 (1986).

[33]Id. at 596–7.

[34]Id. at 597.

[35]Marylou Tousignant and Bill Miller, "Baby K's Mother Gives Her the Prayer That Many Deny She Has," *Washington Post,* October 7, 1994, at A1; E. Haavi Morreim, "Futilitarianism, Exoticare, and Coerced Altruism: The ADA Meets Its Limits," *Seton Hall Law Review* 25:883–926, 1995.

[36]Marylou Tousignant and Bill Miller, "Death of 'Baby K' Leaves a Legacy of Legal Precedent," *Washington Post,* April 7, 1995, at B3.

[37]933 F2d 1037 (DC Cir 1991).

[38]Id. at 1041.

[39]525 US 249.

[40]"EMTALA is a limited 'anti-dumping' statute, not a federal malpractice statute." *Bryan v Rectors and Visitors of the Univ. of Va.,* 95 F3d 349, 351 (4th Cir 1996); see *Correa v Hospital San Francisco,* 69 F3d 1184, 1192 (1st Cir 1995); *Summers v Baptist Med. Ctr. Arkadelphia,* 91 F3d 1132, 1137 (8th Cir 1996) ("So far as we can tell, every court that has considered EMTALA has disclaimed any notion that it creates a general federal cause of action for medical malpractice in emergency rooms."); *Urban v King,* 43 F3d 523, 525 (10th Cir 1994). For an excellent review, see Lynn Healey Scaduto, "The Emergency Medical Treatment and Active Labor Act Gone Astray: A Proposal to Reclaim EMTALA for Its Intended Beneficiaries," *UCLA Law Review* 46:943–82, 1999.

[41]95 F3d 349 (4th Cir 1996).

[42]Id. at 351.

[43]Id.

[44]Id.

[45]86 F3d 885 (9th Cir 1996).

[46]See, for example, *Vickers v Nash Gen. Hosp., Inc.,* 78 F3d 139, 145 (4th Cir 1996) ("The Act does not hold hospitals accountable for failing to stabilize conditions of which they are not aware, or even conditions of which they should have been aware."); *Cleland v Bronson Health Care Group,* 917 F2d 266, 268–9 (6th Cir 1990) ("We hold Congress to its words, that this statute applies to any and all patients. However, we interpret . . . the vague phrase 'emergency medical condition' to mean a condition within the *actual knowledge of the doctors on duty* or those doctors that would have been provided to any paying patient. Since the plaintiffs make no allegations that would allow a finding that either of the statutory duties was breached, we affirm the district court's dismissal of this case." [emphasis added])

[47]Id. at 889.

[48]Id.

[49]Id. at 1134–5.

[50]For an excellent review of this issue, see Julia Ai, "Does EMTALA Apply to Inpatients Located Anywhere in a Hospital?" *Rutgers Law Journal* 32:549, 2001.

[51]416 SE2d 689, 693 (Va 1992).

[52]175 F3d 170 (1st Cir 1999).

[53]*Roberts,* supra, at 253.

[54]Summary of EMTALA conference call with Gloria Frank, HCFA, March 17, 1999. American Hospital Association Web site. Available at: http://www.aha.org/ar/Advocacy/emtala899.asp. Accessed November 11, 2001.

[55]719 So2d 1072 (1998) La App LEXIS 2477 (La App 2d Cir [1998]).

[56]Id. at 1074.

[57]La RS 40:1299.41 et seq.

[58]Id. at 1073–4.

[59]Id. at 1074.

[60]Id. at 1075.

[61]Id. at 1074–5.

[62]Id. at 1075.

[63]Id. at 1076.

[64]Paul R. Helft, Mark Siegler, and John Lantos, "The Rise and Fall of the Futility Movement," *New England Journal of Medicine* 343:293–6, 2000; Steve Heilig, "The Rise and Fall of the Futility Movement" (letter), *New England Journal of Medicine* 343:1575–7, 2000.

[65]James F. Drane and John L. Coulehan, "The Concept of Futility: Patients Do Not Have a Right to Demand Medically Useless Treatment," *Health Progress,* December 1993.

[66]Robert M. Veatch and Carol Mason Spicer, "Futile Care: Physicians Should Not Be Allowed to Refuse to Treat," *Health Progress,* December 1993.

[67]Lawrence J. Schneiderman and Alexander Morgan Capron, "How Can Hospital Futility Policies Contribute to Establishing Standards of Practice?" *Cambridge Quarterly of Healthcare Ethics* 9:524–31, 2000.

[68]American College of Chest Physicians/Society of Critical Care Medicine Consensus Panel, "Ethical and Moral Guidelines for the Initiation, Continuation, and Withdrawal of Intensive Care," *Chest* 97:949–58, 1990; Task Force on Ethics of the Society of Critical Care Medicine, "Consensus Report on the Ethics of Foregoing Life-Sustaining Treatments in the Critically Ill," *Critical Care Medicine* 18:1435–9, 1990; American Thoracic Society Bioethics Task Force, "Withholding and Withdrawing Life-Sustaining Therapy," *Annals of Internal Medicine* 115:478–85, 1991; Emergency Cardiac Care Committee and Subcommittees, American Heart Association, "Guidelines for Cardiopulmonary Resuscitation and Emergency Cardiac Care; Ethical Considerations in Resuscitation," *JAMA* 268:2282–8, 1992.

[69]Society of Critical Care Medicine Ethics Committee, "Triage of Critically Ill Patients," *JAMA* 271:1200–3 at 1202–3.

[70]Steve Heilig, "The Rise and Fall of the Futility Movement" (letter), *New England Journal of Medicine* 343:1575–7, 2000.

[71]For a richly instructive view of the many paradoxes of America's health care system assembled after the demise of the Clinton health care plan, see Henry Aaron, ed. *The Problem That Won't Go Away: Reforming U.S. Health Care Financing.* Washington, DC: The Brookings Institution, 1996.

[72]42 USC §§1395.

[73]Jennifer Steinhauer, "After 5 Years of Fiscal Success, City Public Hospitals Face Deficit," *New York Times,* May 23, 2001.

[74]"Death of the Community Hospital," *The Economist,* January 25, 2001; Sheryl Gay Stolberg, "Washington Is Losing Its Only Public Hospital," *New York Times,* May 7, 2001.

[75]Jack K. Kilcullen, "Groping for the Reins: ERISA, HMO Malpractice, and Enterprise Liability," *American Journal of Law & Medicine* 22:1–44, 1996.

[76]Jennifer Steinhauer, "15 School Health Clinics Scheduled for Closing Get a Reprieve," *New York Times,* June 1, 2001.

Comments From
Paramedical Providers

End-of-Life Care
in the Intensive Care Unit

Gabriele Ford, CCRN

I am sitting in the report room, listening to the charge nurse describe the patients we have in the unit today. For more than 3 years I have worked here as a registered nurse, taking care of a variety of surgical and medical patients, everything but burn patients and transplant recipients. It is 7 A.M. The coffee is strong; I am getting energized.

Today, my patient is a 78-year-old man, here for peritonitis, probably septic. The off-going nurse tells me his history: Parkinson's; lives in a nursing home; two recent admissions for aspiration pneumonia, each time requiring intubation; increasingly unable to swallow food; end-stage renal disease with several years of peritoneal dialysis; now with heightened confusion, fever, a distended abdomen. She rolls her eyes. "He's a full code, too. You get the picture."

Such is the widespread attitude of the staff. We have seen "the picture" many times. A person near the end of his or her life becomes very sick, is admitted to the hospital, takes a turn for the worse, and is transferred into the unit. Now begins the process of diagnostic procedures and treatments. High- and low-tech implements are attached or inserted or clipped and clamped onto the patient's body so that we can measure, weigh, calculate, and otherwise assess all his body functions. Frequently, the patient will have to be sedated or even paralyzed so that he or she will tolerate these investigations and treatments.

I enter the man's room and begin a head-to-toe assessment. Not surprisingly, he is sedated, and when I introduce myself, he looks at me with glazed eyes and begins to get restless. I back off a bit so he will not get agitated. A bilevel positive airway pressure (BiPAP) machine noisily and rhythmically forces air into his nostrils. The helmetlike mask gives the patient the appearance of an astronaut. Bilateral wrist restraints prevent him from pulling off the mask. His temperature is 39.4°C. I notice that his infusions include a sedating agent but no pain control. I make a mental note of that and also plan to remove the wrist restraints if he can be controlled with sedation alone. Blood pressure (BP) 194/94 mm Hg, heart rate 74 beats/min, respiratory rate 14 breaths/min. Nitroglycerin is infusing at 100 μg to lower the BP. Apparently it's not working. His pulses are bounding, and he has severe edema in his extremities. His face is puffy. I listen to the man's lungs and hear a few crackles. Turning to his abdomen, I see a large, distended mound with a dressing over the site where the dialysis catheter was removed. I hear no bowel sounds. A Foley catheter is in place in the urethra—apparently he still makes urine. I notice his groin is red and excoriated. Yeast? Sweat? Sequential compression boots are wrapped tightly around the man's lower legs; this machine is also emitting a rhythmic puffing sound. The cooling option is not on, I see, and I push the button. It might make him a tiny bit more comfortable.

I have now seen the picture. Medications for this patient include intravenous antibiotics, which I hang. I then proceed to give him his heparin shot. His abdomen has several bruises where previous doses were injected subcutaneously.

The primary physician, a nephrologist, is here. I share with him my concerns, and he examines the patient. New orders: stop BiPAP and sedation, oxygen now via nasal prongs, drop a nasogastric (NG) tube, instill contrast medium, take the patient to Computed Tomography (CT) for an abdominal scan. I shudder. It will be a chore to insert a tube into this man's nose—a struggle. Before I can ask anything else, the doctor is gone.

I sigh and gather the material for the NG tube insertion. An aide holds the man's head, tilted forward. We tell him to swallow, swallow, swallow! He thrashes, turning his head from side to side. We hold him tight, and I am relieved that the tube goes down easily. Before I have time to fasten the tube to his nose, a large amount of brownish, thick fluid comes oozing out the end of the tube. The bed is soiled, and some of the fluid has run into the man's armpit. Bother! I hook the tube to the suction machine, and 500 mL of fluid is drained. I place a call to the physician to inform him. "Should we instill contrast?" I ask. Yes, we should. The aide is cleaning the patient, who moans softly when we turn him. I begin to fill the patient's tender abdomen with contrast. Then we prepare for the trip to CT. I have to call his wife to inform her and get permission. Luckily she is at home.

"Oh," she says, "he has had so many tests already. I hate to see him put through more. What was his potassium this morning?" She has become wise to the jargon and procedures. Her schedule revolves around the hospital, and she visits every day from 10 A.M. to 3 P.M. It's her job.

"So you don't want your husband to have this test?" I ask, hopefully.

"Ah, well, go ahead," she says. We're going.

We transfer the patient onto the scanner table. A stream of diarrhea smears the sheets, the bed, the scanner. The smell is terrible, but time is precious, and we cover both it and the patient up, tighten a Velcro belt around his chest, and shove him into the scanner. He mumbles some incoherent phrases.

As soon as the test concludes, we have to get out of the room because another patient is waiting. I find myself in the elevator with the patient, portable monitoring equipment, pumps, and a terrible odor. On our return to the room, I hook up the NG tube, and a huge amount of fluid drains. I think it must be time for a pain shot for the poor man. I'll medicate him before we wrestle with his large, swollen body to wash him up.

Another doctor arrives. He reads the chart for a very long time and then announces that the patient is infected. The doctor wants everything cultured. "Get a sputum sample from him, blood cultures times two, daily complete blood count, mini chem, get Pharmacy to give me a printout of what antibiotics he's been on and for how long." He's gone.

Meanwhile, the patient's wife arrives. She plants herself in the room—obviously has a regular spot. She tells me her husband needs dialysis and she wants to know the CT results. She points to the brown NG fluid. I explain that his stomach is not working right. I point out his mental status, and she informs me that he is "usually pretty with it." The speech therapist arrives to perform a swallow evaluation. I tell her I don't think it's appropriate right now and request that she ask the patient's wife how her husband has been eating recently.

The nephrologist returns with a Quinton catheter kit, and I hold the patient still so the nephrologist can puncture the femoral vein and insert the large-bore catheter. "Make sure we don't lose it," he says at the conclusion of the procedure. I will try to position the man with his right leg fairly straight; he now has yet another gadget to prevent movement and natural positioning. The patient didn't flinch when the lidocaine syringe was poked into his groin. He seems detached, almost like a tortured person who has removed himself from the source of pain. The renal doctor informs me in parting that the CT scan showed some pockets and he will ask Radiology to drain them. I reposition the patient; time for a shot of morphine and maybe some lorazepam.

Another doctor arrives. It's the surgeon who removed the dialysis catheter, just checking up. The patient looks comfortable now—no traces of the insults and calamities that befell him during the morning. The puff boots are back in place, the drains are draining, the cultures are cooking, drugs and oxygen are finding their way into his insides. On his last visit, the nephrologist wrote orders to stop the nitroglycerin and start a sodium nitroprusside infusion to control the patient's BP. We need a new intravenous infusion. I look over the patient's arms and notice a few sites where he was poked for arterial blood gas analysis.

Suddenly two technicians and a nurse show up. "We're from Radiology," they announce. I'd forgotten. The patient is turned just so, his abdomen is exposed, his arms are fastened. With a perfunctory "We're going to take a look inside your belly," they drop a mound of gel onto his abdomen so that the ultrasound probe can glide across his skin. The radiologist arrives, and with the help of the sonographer, he finds two pockets of fluid and sticks a catheter into each. Some yellowish fluid drains into a vacuum bottle. Some is kept for samples. Outside the room, the patient's wife is having a conversation with the social worker. They discuss the patient's living situation in the long-term-care facility.

It is 3 P.M. I am exhausted. The patient is alternately restless or sedated. He talks occasionally, but I cannot understand him. He can't tell me, but I sense he is in pain, if only from having all that equipment wrapped and taped and stitched onto his skin. I have removed his wrist restraints, but during all the procedures, he had to be held down so much that he might as well have been restrained. I feel terrible that he has been so manhandled today for tests and procedures. He seems not to care. He doesn't even react when his monitor alarm goes off loudly—atrial fibrillation! I can't believe it! His BP doesn't change, he seems unaware, his breathing is unchanged— but how long can he sustain a heart rate of 180 beats/min? I call the nephrologist, and he orders digitalis.

I think about the procession of doctors and other health care professionals who had contact with my patient today. Did any of them make a difference in his status? He is still very febrile and restless, with failing lungs and kidneys and now a racing heart. He is swollen in bed, unable to turn himself; areas of his body are bruised or raw. He has been subjected to painful and undignified procedures. He endured them. I have diligently carried out the orders, like a soldier. I did not want to hurt him, but I certainly inflicted pain on him in following the orders. Everything looks good on paper. We treated him, spared no expense, and enlisted the help of a large number of doctors, nurses, technicians, therapists, a dietitian, a social worker, and many unseen workers. His wife is content that we are treating him. She is eager, involved in his "care." His doctors are aggressively seeking to turn around his downslide. The patient moans or alternately slips into a blissful sedated state. The respiratory therapist will connect him to the

BiPAP machine again, for overnight. Restraints, the discomfort of air forced into his lungs, sedation—the routine continues. Arterial blood gas analysis in the morning, chest X-ray, blood draws, morning rounds.

I think to myself that somebody needs to bring up the topic of futile care. Are we healing this man, or are we slowing his death from sepsis or multiple organ failure? We need one doctor who will assume charge of his care and evaluate the appropriateness of treatments. We need this doctor to have a frank conversation with the patient's wife. Perhaps the nephrologist will call one more consultation in the morning and ask the intensivist to assume overall care. It would be a step in the right direction. I will suggest it, citing the need for involvement of the intensivist for pulmonary management.

I have the next 4 days off. When I return to work, I am assigned to another department for 2 days. The next time I am in the unit, I inquire about "the picture." Did we control his situation? Did he respond to the procedures? What's his status? The charge nurse tells me that he didn't tolerate dialysis, and after several more days of decline, they "let him go." The nurses in the report room are unfazed. We have to be, or we couldn't do it again tomorrow.

Selected Bibliography

Cassell EJ: The principles of the Belmont report revisited. How have respect for persons, beneficence, and justice been applied to clinical medicine? Hastings Cent Rep 2000;30:12–21.

Cogliano JF: The medical futility controversy: bioethical implications for the critical care nurse. Crit Care Nurs Q 1999;22:81–8.

Advanced Medical Technology and End of Life
A Respiratory Care Practitioner's Perspective

David H. Walker, MA, RRT, RCP

I have had the good fortune to work in intensive care medicine as a respiratory care practitioner for 33 years. During that time, I have seen the introduction of new technology, mostly from manufacturers of mechanical ventilators. Each new generation of mechanical ventilators has been touted as providing perfect treatment to patients with acute or chronic respiratory failure. However, even with the latest new ventilator platform, even with flashing lights displayed on a breath-by-breath basis, patients still die.

Currently, we are ventilating a 70-year-old man with obvious multiple organ failure that includes severe abdominal distention, which is compromising the patient's gas exchange ($PaCO_2$ of 70 mm Hg). The man has been receiving mechanical ventilation for 2 weeks and underwent a tracheotomy yesterday, because the intensive care unit (ICU) physician believes that all patients should have tracheotomy tubes placed after 1 week of intubation. The patient is so agitated that placing the tracheotomy tube was probably a good idea; it might prevent damage and irritation from the endotracheal tube. In addition to being agitated, our patient is also very confused and combative, so much so that the nurse and I are almost completed exhausted after wrestling with him for 3 hours during our shift.

This week we have a new attending physician who does not know the patient very well and does not seem very interested in gathering pertinent clinical information from the nurse or me. Yesterday we were using pressure control ventilation and the patient was very comfortable, even after placement of the tracheotomy tube. This morning, during rounds, the ICU doctor tells us that it is time to start weaning the patient and orders synchronized intermittent mandatory ventilation (SIMV). I immediately suggest to the physician that the patient will not tolerate breathing with SIMV, given his abdominal distention. The physician is somewhat annoyed that I have questioned his decision. I direct his attention to the pressure-volume loops displayed on the ventilator's monitoring screen. The graphics clearly demonstrate that the patient's work of breathing has increased since the switch to SIMV. I immediately notice that my comments are not particularly important to the physician, but he does listen to my concerns as he writes the orders in the patient's chart. After signing the orders, the physician tells me that he does not know the details of lung mechanics monitoring but he thinks that the data are not accurate and are certainly not a valid reason for not ventilating the patient with SIMV. My first reaction is that I have been working in intensive care longer than this physician has been alive, but I quickly tell myself that the physician is in charge and has the final word in patient care decisions.

After I return from lunch, the patient's agitation and confusion is so bad that he is trying to get out of bed while at the same time complaining of shortness of breath. The nurse and I think we should call the physician and request additional sedation to keep the patient from injuring himself. So the nurse pages the physician, who responds within just a few minutes and orders immediate chest radiography and blood gas analysis. Fifteen minutes later, the X-ray technician brings the developed film to the bedside, while the nurse writes down the blood gas measurements on her flow sheet.

The ICU physician enters a couple of minutes later, reviews the X-ray and blood gas measurements, and requests that I increase positive end-expiratory pressure (PEEP) from 6 to 8 cm H_2O, because PaO_2 is decreasing and $PaCO_2$ is increasing. Respectfully, I inform the physician that the patient's abdominal girth has increased 3 cm since early this morning and that is the reason for the poor gas exchange. In addition, the patient's respiratory rate has increased from 16 to 30 breaths/min since we switched to SIMV. The physician tells me that the patient is developing acute respiratory distress syndrome and that the abdominal distention has nothing to do with the loss of oxygenation or the increased $PaCO_2$. So I increase PEEP to 8 cm H_2O while the physician observes the pulse oximeter for an increase in oxygen saturation. In the meantime, the patient becomes even more agitated and pulls out two intravenous lines, although the nurse and I are trying our best to calm him.

We now have to suction the patient, which only agitates him even more, to the point that I am really afraid that he may dislodge his tracheotomy tube. The physician finally orders additional sedation, to include neuromuscular blockade. Now that the patient is paralyzed, I ask the physician if it is OK to switch the ventilator to pressure control mode, but he insists that increasing the SIMV rate is the best strategy. So now I increase the SIMV rate from 6 to 15 breaths/min, while the physician requests that I increase

PEEP to 15 cm H_2O because oxygen saturation has not improved.

As I slowly increase PEEP, I notice that at 12 cm H_2O, the pressure-volume loop has a definite overdistension pattern. I immediately inform the physician, who is listening to the patient's breath sounds. The physician tells me that the lung sounds have improved and to increase PEEP to 15 cm H_2O. I do so, and 30 minutes later the nurse tells me that urine output has decreased by 50% and the patient's blood pressure is very labile. I know now that we are doing harm to this poor patient, and there seems nothing to do except watch and hope for the best. Three hours later, the patient's gas exchange has not improved. He is now developing metabolic acidosis along with his respiratory acidosis. The physician enters, making evening rounds, and tells the nurse that he wants to place a Swan-Ganz catheter to assist with fluids management but that he will wait for the night physician to make the final decision. It is at this point that I realize that even with the use of the most advanced technology in the ICU, patients still die—and not always in a dignified manner. In fact, these technologies may prolong the suffering of critically ill patients.

Before I prepare for report to the oncoming respiratory care practitioner, I log on to the Internet to review the current published research on ventilating patients with multiple organ failure. Because we have online access to the journals in the hospital's library, I can review entire articles after I find them listed in MEDLINE. I soon discover that for every article that presents one point of view, there is at least one other documenting that there is a completely different way to produce the same clinical outcome.

Just as I finish reviewing an online article, the patient's daughter comes up to me and asks how her father is doing today. I tell her that he is not quite as good as yesterday but that she should talk to the physician to find out the details. She then tells me that she has done her own research on the Internet and believes that we are not treating her father according to current literature. At this time, the nurse comes to join us and assures the daughter that we are doing everything possible for her father. The daughter then tells us that she wants everything done for her father but that she does not want him to suffer. Both the nurse and I inform her of the day's events and what the physicians plan to do if they decide to place the Swan-Ganz catheter later in the evening.

In the meantime, the unit's medical director comes into the room and inquires about the patient's condition. The medical director is very knowledgeable about mechanical ventilation and associated lung mechanics monitoring. I point out the pressure-volume loop as well as the decreased urine output following the increase in PEEP to 15 cm H_2O. Our director then asks for my impression, and I suggest decreasing PEEP and switching the ventilator to pressure control mode. He agrees with me, and the changes are made. Two hours later, as I am preparing to go home, the nurse tells me that the patient's urine output has increased and his blood pressure has improved. At the same time, the night physician asks the nurse and me what the day physician's rationale was for placing a Swan-Ganz catheter, given the patient's improvement. We cannot answer his question, but we are very glad for his insight.

The next morning, I arrive at the ICU to find the patient's wife and daughter at his bedside, looking very grim, to say the least. They tell me that the physicians are considering exploratory abdominal surgery and are asking for their consent to schedule the surgery later in the morning. Suddenly, green ooze pours from around the tracheotomy stoma and runs down the patient's neck and onto the pillowcase. Both wife and daughter decide that surgery would only prolong the man's suffering and take away his dignity during his last days alive. Six hours later, our patient dies from a sudden cardiac arrest. In accordance with the family's wishes, we did not perform cardiopulmonary resuscitation.

To prepare the ventilator for cleaning, I must strip it down (remove the tubing and humidifier) and quickly wipe off the entire machine. I then call Central Supply to request a more thorough cleaning. After the Central Supply technician wheels the ventilator away, my supervisor pages me to remind me of an in-service meeting on a new ventilator that we are currently evaluating. When I sit down at the meeting with my coffee and two donuts (supplied by the ventilator sales representative), I ask myself, "Where are the physicians? Shouldn't they understand how this new ventilator works?" I also wonder, "Will this new ventilator really help critically ill patients or just prolong their agony?"

Selected Bibliography

Cardiopulmonary education clinical resources Web site. Available at: http://home.earthlink.net/~firstbreath. Accessed October 28, 2001.

Diehl J-L, Isabey D, Desmarais G, et al: Physiological effects of alveolar, tracheal, and "standard" pressure supports. J Appl Physiol 87:428–37, 1999.

Landro L: Information technology could revolutionize the practice of medicine. But not anytime soon. Wall Street Journal. June 25, 2001:R14.

Neumann P, Berglund JE, Mondéjar EF, et al: Dynamics of lung collapse and recruitment during prolonged breathing in porcine lung injury. J Appl Physiol 85:1533–43, 1998.

Polkey MI, Hamnegård C-H, Hughes PD, et al: Influence of acute lung volume change on contractile properties of human diaphragm. J Appl Physiol 85:1322–8, 1998.

The Role of the Internet in Health Care. Ernst and Young 1997. Available at: http://www.ey.com.

Medical Futility

Leslie Beckhart Jenal, JD

All people suffer, but a person who suffers well may find that his or her suffering is wrapped in a promise. A person who suffers well, who makes his or her suffering meaningful, may ultimately transform that suffering into a source of deeper meaning in life. The only value of suffering lies in its transformative power.

If suffering—whether physical pain, apprehension, anxiety, fear, loss, or feelings of abandonment—is an inevitable consequence of purposeful medical treatment, then a patient may find meaning in it. But suffering that is a consequence of medically futile treatment will never be meaningful, and not only because of the meaninglessness of the treatment itself. Futile medical treatment causes meaningless suffering because implicit within the concept of medical futility is the idea that the patient's physiological life is worth more than what makes the patient human and gives his or her life meaning. As Viktor Frankl[1] wrote, when a person's suffering is meaningless, in the "bitter fight for self-preservation he may forget his human dignity and become no more than an animal."

The most critical time for a patient or family member to exercise decisional autonomy is when a physician has suggested that a medical treatment may be futile. In this context, a patient or family member does not exercise autonomy effectively by selecting from a menu of medical treatments. That person exercises autonomy effectively when he or she evaluates the essential medical facts (the patient's condition, including the extent of suffering, and the reasonably likely beneficial and adverse consequences of any treatment under consideration) with reference to the values that consistently have given meaning to the patient's life. If a patient or family member refuses to accept that a treatment is futile, he or she either does not understand the medical facts or is referring to the wrong set of values. As a chaplain, I support patients and families as they struggle to evaluate treatment in light of patients' values.

Many people do not understand basic medical terms, or, worse, they base their understanding on what they have seen on television. A physician

can help a patient or a patient's family understand the basic facts by providing qualitative information (preferably using visual descriptions) as well
as quantitative data. For example, a physician may describe cardiopulmonary resuscitation (CPR) in visual terms to a family member who is
resisting a do-not-resuscitate order. The physician may set the scene by
pointing out the number of participants involved; the type and amount of
force typically used during compressions, and the associated risk of broken
bones; and the means by which electric shocks are applied to the heart. He
or she also may provide quantitative data such as the approximate rate of
survival to discharge for patients who undergo in-hospital CPR (particularly
patients not in coronary care units, if that is relevant) and the amount of time
that a patient may be deprived of oxygen before developing brain damage.
In my experience, a family member who knows what CPR looks like and
understands the likelihood of its success in the patient's case will become
more comfortable with a do-not-resuscitate order.

A family member who is unfamiliar with critical care practices may
believe that a patient is resting comfortably when he or she is actually in
pain and anxious unless sedated. If this family member demands futile treatment, it may be because he or she lacks information about the patient's
medications, particularly those prescribed for pain, anxiety, and fear and
those prescribed to enable the patient to tolerate a ventilator.

Every patient and family member who makes a decision is responsible
for gathering the information he or she requires. The reality, however, is that
many patients and family members fail to understand the facts because they
do not ask questions. Some are intimidated by the physician involved, or
fear that asking the physician a question will offend him or her, and many
are in the throes of emotional shock or anticipatory grief. A common
behavior of family members struggling to make or rationalize a decision is
to lock onto a single phrase spoken by the physician and repeat the phrase
over and over, its meaning often becoming lost. A patient or family member
may also lock onto an initial-version or provisional diagnosis implying a
reasonably favorable prognosis, despite its having been revised or even
discarded. In both cases, the behavior is generally kept within the family and
the physician may not be aware of it. As a chaplain and trusted visitor at the
patient's bedside, I do not believe that I breach confidentiality when I alert a
physician that he or she may need to reinforce an earlier explanation.

On the other hand, the fault lies with physicians when a patient or
family member receives conflicting information. The most common example occurs when a specialist reports to a patient or family that the patient
has recovered from the condition for which the specialist was consulted, but

the specialist neglects to place this information within the general context of the patient's entire condition. In the worst cases, the patient and his or her family have already come to terms with the futility of further treatment but are persuaded otherwise when the patient's physicians flatly contradict each other. Two or more nurses may also confuse family members when they relate the same information about the patient's condition but use different terminology.

I once worked with the family of a patient who attempted suicide by shooting himself through the mouth with a shotgun. A fist-sized portion of his brain was exposed to the open air on the left side of his forehead. The paramedics reported that he had left a large amount of his brain in the ambulance. The patient was ventilated in the emergency department. After being informed by the emergency attending physician that the patient's prognosis was abysmal, the family took the initiative and approached the medical staff about donating his organs. The patient was moved to intensive care and was tested as a non-heart-beating donor. A consulting neuro-surgeon arrived and suggested to the family that with surgery, the patient might "recover." He also told the family that if the patient were his son, "in case something does happen, I'd want to know that I did everything possible for him." Immediately after the neurosurgeon's visit, every family member present was prepared to agree that the surgery should take place. They told me that the neurosurgeon's statement "I'd want to know that I did every-thing possible for him" did far more to persuade them to agree to surgery than his suggestion that recovery might be possible. The lesson here is clear. To many family members and patients, the physician's opinion of the ethics of the case ("If I were you, I would go for it and give him a little more time") is just as powerful, if not more powerful, than his or her medical judgment. In this case, however, the family ultimately recognized that the neurosurgeon's personal values conflicted with their own and agreed to withdrawal of life support. The patient died peacefully.

Finally, it can be difficult for a physician to debunk incorrect infor-mation. Much of this information is anecdotal and irrelevant: "When Aunt Mary had cancer, they gave her radiation and now look, she's 80 and she's just fine now" or "I don't think that doctor's right. Oprah had a lady on the other day whose doctor wanted to pull the plug and she's fine now." Some information is from the press: "What about this new drug I read about in *Time* magazine?" or "I read that B_{12} complex works really well for cancer" or even "I heard about a new type of diet for cancer where you eat nothing but soybeans." A family may have great difficulty accepting that a treatment is medically futile if a family member who is powerful in the decision-making process is the source of the misinformation. A family member may also contribute misinformation he or she believes to be accurate, in an effort to wrest control from the physician or to jockey for a more powerful role in the family's decision making. A patient may also express denial by citing misinformation.

As a chaplain, I am more directly involved when a patient's emotional state prevents the patient from discerning his or her true values or when family members fail to respect the patient's values. For example, I have met many Christian patients who are less afraid of death than of what comes after death. Their image of God is harsh: God is punishing, retributive, and even vindictive, and they expect a harsh judgment. However, if a patient who is afraid of judgment is invited to tell his or her story or to review his or her life, the patient inevitably will disclose or confess whatever it is that he or she believes is sinful, and that person may greatly benefit if he or she is able to accept God's forgiveness. An 80-year-old woman once disclosed to me that as a child, she had experienced serious sexual abuse at the hands of her brother and her mother. She considered her innocent response to the abuse to be a horrible sin, and she said that her guilt had "ruined" her marriage and her relationship with her children. Once she was reassured that she was not at fault and that God certainly would forgive her for damaging her relationships, she was able to accept a change in her living situation that she had refused many times before. A patient may also reveal that he or she cannot die before finishing a task or reconciling with a loved one. We know how a patient in the last hours of life may seem to wait until he or she has permission to die, but a patient who has not yet reached that point may accept that treatment is futile more easily if he or she receives permission to die and leave unfinished tasks.

It frustrates me, as well as the physicians involved, when a patient consistently repeats that he or she wants to die but demands that everything be done, or refuses to decide what amount of treatment he or she wants, or changes his or her mind frequently, or vacillates between demanding futile treatment and demanding euthanasia. This patient may well fear that death entails intolerable pain and indignity, despite his or her physician's assurances and descriptions of hospice treatment available. Essentially, the patient is extending aggressive treatment and suffering indignity, if not pain, instead of accepting the care that could assure him or her a comfortable and dignified death.

The task for a family member of an incompetent patient is complex. Ideally, that family member sets aside his or her own values in order to advise the physician what the patient would do if he or she were competent.

Often a family member must be assured that his or her task is only to relate information about the patient's values, and not to determine by himself or herself whether the patient lives or dies.

Inevitably, the dynamics of the family affect discussions about the futility of treatment. For one thing, it is important to recognize that the death of the patient will not have the same impact on all family members, and the patient's place in the family structure may not be obvious. For example, the death of a patient who has been a long-time substance abuser may be a relief to the patient's mother but a loss to his or her siblings, or vice versa. In addition, it may be difficult to determine who makes the decisions in the family. The decision maker may be the patient's mother for legal purposes; the patient's grandmother, who raised him or her, from a moral perspective; and the patient's strong-willed younger brother in actuality. Finally, the stress of the patient's illness also may fracture the family according to old conflicts or may create new conflicts and alliances. A family's cultural tradition may contribute to internal conflict, particularly if the younger generation is significantly more acculturated than the older, or conflict may arise because family members have differing religious affiliations or differing levels of faith.

It is also immensely frustrating to me when family members focus on their own needs instead of the patient's. Very frequently, a family member will demand futile treatment for a patient by saying, "I need to know that I did everything," requesting the futile treatment in order to meet his or her emotional needs, at the expense of the patient's suffering. In other cases, a family member who feels guilty over a past conflict with the patient may demand futile treatment because the family member fears feeling even more guilt when the patient dies. Some family members also may demand further treatment in the hope that the patient will regain consciousness long enough for them to reconcile past differences. In any case, a meaningful reconciliation is impossible if the patient is not competent, and the family member should be encouraged instead to make the kindest decision.

Family members with latent psychological needs also request futile treatment. For example, the daughter of a patient who had abandoned her as an infant refused to accept that treatment for her mother was futile. She believed that her mother would be discharged and that she could take her home to care for her, perhaps in an effort to buy her mother's love. The daughter decided on her own to request withdrawal of treatment after she had an opportunity to share her feelings over a period of days.

A family member may refuse to accept limitations on a patient's care if the patient's death itself is complicated by religious or emotional factors.

For example, I worked with the Roman Catholic grandmother of a patient who had attempted to commit suicide. Although the grandmother knew that the patient's death was imminent, she persistently prevented his mother from agreeing to withdrawal from life support. The grandmother believed that her grandson had committed a mortal sin by attempting suicide and that God would send him to hell. She was reassured that the Catholic Church teaches that God is more loving than he is judgmental and that he considers all mitigating circumstances when judging persons who commit suicide. Once the grandmother was able to trust that God would forgive her grandson in light of his long history of depression, she agreed that life support should be withdrawn.[2]

Sometimes a patient or family member will fall back on familiar statements that reject the medical facts entirely. For example, the statements "God does not want him to hurt" and "God wants to cure him" may well be true but are nevertheless inconsistent with the reality that God permits people to suffer and die all the time. "Medical science does not have all the answers" is inconsistent with a contemporaneous demand for futile treatment. "Life and death is in God's hands," generally used to denigrate the medical profession and to oppose the withdrawal of treatment, may also mean the converse—that an inappropriate use of medical technology will obstruct God's purposes if it prevents the patient from dying in his or her proper time. The only recourse against statements such as these is to reemphasize the facts—that the patient's condition is irreversible and that he or she is suffering—and to suggest that the patient has suffered enough.

Finally, many patients and families express their literal belief in miracles. Although it might be argued that God does not intervene to suspend the laws of physics and that it is narcissistic to believe otherwise, a belief in miracles must nevertheless be respected, particularly where it is integral to a person's religious faith.[3] A belief in miracles, however, need not preclude a discussion about the futility of treatment. For example, when the belief is presented as a test ("If I have enough faith, God will grant me a miracle"), it may be effective to suggest a time limit or series of time limits, after which the patient's condition will be reassessed. It is important to keep in mind that because the person who believes he or she is being tested may believe he or she has failed in loving God if the miracle fails to appear, the person may benefit from a chaplain's support. Another example is where a family member believes that the patient must remain biologically alive "long enough for God to have a chance to work a miracle," a belief I have heard more frequently expressed in neonatal than in adult intensive care units. One effective approach is to reinforce the sovereignty and omnipotence of God, perhaps with scripture passages referring to the raising of the dead, with care being taken to avoid challenging the family's underlying faith.

I believe that all people are created in the image of God. I also believe that meaningless suffering—which preserves the mere fact of a person's physiological life but sacrifices what gives his or her life meaning and darkens the spark of the divine in him or her—is an affront to God. Therefore, it is my duty not only as a chaplain but as a human being to prevent patients and families from perpetuating meaningless suffering. Theology, religion, faith, and spirituality can be powerful weapons. I confess that I am sometimes tempted to use them offensively and coerce people to do the right thing. Fortunately, I have found that most people need just a gentle touch before they recognize the truth, and most are just good enough to act on the truth when they try.

Notes

[1] Viktor E. Frankl, *Man's Search for Meaning*. 4th ed. Translated by Ilse Lasch. Boston, MA: Beacon, 1992.

[2] A chaplain may consult with a minister of the appropriate denomination in any case that hinges on a theological issue unique to that denomination.

[3] For example, a person who is a Pentecostal or charismatic Christian, or even a believer in some New Age spiritualities, may express a literal belief in miracles.

Afterword

David Crippen, MD

> Liberty means responsibility. That is why most men dread it.
> —George Bernard Shaw, *Man and Superman*

In a perfect world, there would be a perfect balance of resources. Medical care provision would form a balance of resources for the patient's benefit—a balance between what the populace needs and what it desires. In this imperfect world, there is a balance of contentiousness—a balance between what the populace and what the administrators of its resources find authoritative and binding. An ecosystem of immanent domain and individual rights is held in delicate balance by multifarious forces. In health care delivery, there is a delicate balance also between the ability to fulfill consumer desires, and consumer needs. That balance is maintained by poorly defined, free-floating forces. Society is preoccupied with the individual rights of citizenry, a preoccupation bordering on obsession. In its haste to ensure that the rights of individuals are protected, society frequently ignores the concept of greater good. That is why handguns are sold to citizens and why, to avoid erroneous conviction of 1 innocent, 10 guilty are let go. Society is willing to accept the very strong potential for future harm, in order to protect immediate individual autonomy. Any untoward consequences resulting from individual rights' being protected are unfortunate but not unfair.

Medical care that serves only to preserve vital signs of dying patients with no chance for improvement happens in health care provision. Health care consumers have a strong incentive to demand everything they can get, because the potential stakes are high. They have been told by the media that the health care industry can do miracles, and they want miracles. To them, giving up has no potential to obtain even marginal benefit. "Doing everything" can sometimes gain some ground. And miracles occasionally happen. To an increasing number of patients or surrogates, any decision that contradicts their hearts' desires is unacceptable, and they reject it. To them, it is a physician's role to turn their desires into realities, not dictate paternalistic dogma. Long shots are popular in the media. Women with advanced breast cancer play well when they sue their health maintenance organizations for unproven treatments that might increase their life spans a few months at a phenomenal cost. It is socially acceptable for "someone" to pay for such care, but it is not socially acceptable for the expense to be passed along to the rest of the health maintenance organization clientele. People routinely go on talk shows to relate stories about how doctors forecasted doom and gloom for a moribund patient. They persisted, waiting for a miracle, and beat the odds. In the words of one tearful woman on a representative late-night talk show: "Don't let them talk you out of following your heart."

But following one's heart has consequences for the majority of patients who do not beat the odds, and those consequences do not necessarily involve wasted resources. Cost is not much of an issue on either side. Patients rarely have to underwrite the costs of intensive care, and there is little convincing evidence that money spent on patently futile care affects provision for the rest of the population. Most critical care physicians are willing to expend even the most scarce resources over a reasonable period for even the most moribund patient. But when success is not quickly forthcoming, those consequences can be profoundly different than previous hopeful expectations. They can involve making innocents profoundly uncomfortable for the sake of wildly speculative long shots. Admitting patients with long-standing chronic hemodynamic and metabolic diseases for multiple episodes of decompensation poorly amenable to resuscitation is not a big problem for their families if doing so is their hearts' desire. The patient looks very comfortable there in that intensive care unit (ICU) bed (sedated and restrained). That ventilator is certainly doing its job. That dialysis machine is doing a great job of cleaning up blood volume. And dressings are changed daily on all the decomposing areas. The patient does not look uncomfortable at all. This is certainly easier on families than having to deal with such unpleasantness as stopping life support. Families do not like to take responsibility for decisions that directly result in death. All these things are here to keep people alive.

But there is accumulating evidence that arrested death spirals followed by maintenance of life-in-death via machines can make patients profoundly uncomfortable and sometimes even promote genuine agony. These patients are not able to communicate that agony, because of distorted cerebral integration and sedation regimens that provide only restraint and a false sense of comfort. The patients' surrogates are allowed to misread the situation because their sincere belief in the potential for a miracle clouds their ordinarily sound judgment. And physicians allow these judgments because they are as afraid of being labeled paternalistic as they are of actually being so.

In terms of end-of-life care, physicians usually allow patients and surrogates to define what "everything" in "doing everything" means, and then give them the option of choosing all the technical implementations of "everything" from a laundry list thoughtfully provided for their convenience. Instead of clarifying their options, physicians give them more technical routes to implement flights of fantasy. And as a final insult, physicians allow these unfortunate patients to undergo the useless gesture of cardiopulmonary resuscitation (CPR), unwilling to buck the bad judgment of surrogates lulled into complacency on the basis of false hopes.

Somewhere along the continuum of critical care practice, critical care physicians perceived that do-not-resuscitate concepts need to be more structured. They thought that patients and their families requested fruitless end-of-life care because they did not understand the options. Specifically, they did not understand that there are "better" options than ritual CPR and maintaining warm cadavers in acute care hospital areas just because resources are available. More specifically, they did not appreciate the productive option of maintenance of comfort measures instead of invasive manipulations tantamount to battery in ICU beds. If physicians could simply get patients and their families to understand the consequences of the laundry list of options available at the end of life, they would then be informed consumers and choose the right ones.

Critical care physicians made a tactical mistake. Because of their fear of paternalism, they presented these options as if they had equal weight and then asked patients and families to choose what they desired, not what training and experience dictated was right for the situation. And critical care physicians also gave the impression that if everything was not done, they were doing less than everything and did not realize the subliminal connotations of what they were doing.

"So, Mrs. Jones, your husband is dying. Here are the options you have. Would you like us to do everything we can to make him get better? Of course you would. So here is a list of things we can do if you would like us to do everything: CPR, vasoactive drug therapy, mechanical ventilation, dialysis, extracorporeal membrane oxygenation, heart and lung transplantations. But if you don't want us to do everything, we'll give up and just let your husband die."

Mrs. Jones says, "Well, you have made it plain that there are only two options: doing everything and doing less than everything. I think I owe it to my husband to do everything, so I'll just check off each of these things that imply everything is being done, and we'll hope for the best."

And so it went.

The informed-consent pendulum is slowly swinging in terms of end-of-life care. Critical care physicians are slowly coming around to avoid structuralizing end-of-life care any more than necessary, because of unintended consequences. Bereaved and sometimes hysterical relatives of moribund patients will grab at anything within reach that suggests the remotest hope. And current ethical dogma encourages them on the basis of inviolate individual freedom without prudent consideration of the consequences. Even if I state that dialysis and vasoactive drugs will not be of any use, in the same breath I am stating that these things are on the laundry list and they are available. If they do not work, why should surrogates have access to them? If they do not work, why are they even brought up? They should not be. There is an implied trust that highly trained and experienced critical care physicians have a reasonable idea how to deal with critically ill patients and are capable of doing what is reasonable on every level. If I am trusted to make acute resuscitation decisions without specific consent, it follows that making medically appropriate end-of-life decisions is part of my expertise.

I say that everything that is reasonable will be done at all levels of care. I do not specifically say that unreasonable things will not be done, but I think that is heavily implied. More is not always better. A clearer view of the trees does not necessarily define the forest. So if I never specifically state that CPR or any other specific treatment is anywhere in the care plan, I am not obligated to give it on demand. If I avoid even mentioning dialysis as an option, I avoid a fight over whether it should be given as a panic gesture to maintain a "hope" fantasy. And when the patient dies in an inevitable death spiral, I tell the family that we did everything that was reasonable, not necessarily possible. The fewer details of what is possible, the better. Patients and their families want to know that everything reasonable is being done, but they have no need to know about things that are not effective. Reasonability is implied in the package.

Readers of this book have been exposed to a multidisciplinary discourse of opinions from a multinational panel of working health care providers in the critical care arena. Readers have seen that everyone has an opinion, and even though those opinions are shaped by locality, the fundamental thrust is the same: to do the right thing for sick patients; to maximize their benefit and minimize their detriment by accurately matching resources to need. The ability to reach that effective level of care depends on who is in charge of it.

The contributors to this book have elucidated the problems that surrogates cause if they demand inappropriate end-of-life care. In discussing these problems, we may have implied that surrogates demand this care on the basis of sociopathic arrogance and manipulation. In reality, there are such patients and surrogates, but they are few in number. The majority of patients and surrogates who demand inappropriate care have not been effectively counseled by their health care providers. They demand such care because they are allowed to build expectations on emotion and not reality, and because many times their physicians understand as little as they do about end-of-life care. The primary caregiver has perhaps known the patient for years, has an emotional investment, and has earned the family's confidence. The provider may buy into remote long shots for a lot of the same reasons that his or her patients do. And then a critical care consultant arrives—a specialist who has invested little in long-term family dynamics and has not earned the family's trust. This pretender may bring up emotionally painful options, with the result that formerly free-floating hostility finds a logical destination.

Accordingly, families can perceive conflicting end-of-life signals from multiple levels of providers. One physician whom the patient's family has just met is stating that restraint is in order. The long-time friend and physician is advising that a more aggressive approach is appropriate. These types of conflicts add to the bewilderment of the family and give family members the incentive to resolve the conflict by taking the most comfortable path. Such situations can place the critical care physician at odds with the family and other physicians. Therefore, for this any many other reasons, it seems desirable to ensure that critical care specialists are deeply rooted in ICUs as medical directors and department heads. This ensures their authority and visibility in dealing with all ICU patients on an ongoing basis and permits their specific end-of-life expertise to permeate effective patient and family education. In a heterogeneous health care provision plan, the physician team must have an equally unified and authoritative front.

There should be a balance. But when there cannot be a balance because of fundamental incompatibilities, there must be a consensus that favors patient comfort. If the decisions of patients and their families are given disproportionate weight, physicians will reach a consensus only with their consent, and their consent will function independently from clinical realities. Physicians' progress in supporting effective ICU end-of-life issues depends on how successfully they can modify the disproportionate share of consumer clout that has resulted from current paternalistic concepts. If consumers are in charge, they have the potential to demand resource allocation that is cost-effective only to them, and they may force physicians to use their expertise and training to perpetrate useless and prolonged discomfort. If consumers are in charge, they have the potential to bring life-in-death discomfort on the elderly and infirm for the slightest of long-shot benefit. If they are in charge, they will tell ICU directors when the elderly and infirm can have beds and how long they can occupy them. That is where the paternalism argument is going. It is not an argument about autonomy. It is an argument about balance, or the lack thereof. It is about the ability of physicians to reach a meaningful consensus of benefit without necessarily obtaining consent.

I will conclude by presenting the thrust of this book:

- Not surprisingly, the global village of critical care providers is very consistent in its ability to provide high-quality medical care to critically ill patients. The United States stands out for its tolerance of patients' dictating the terms of critical care provision at an exorbitant cost, but there is no convincing evidence that end-of-life care in the United States is better than that in the rest of the global village.

- The ritual of death in America is no longer a simple, home-based affair in which citizens die in the bosom of their families. It has changed into a technological exercise in which ICUs are used as high-tech hospices. A consumer society has developed to support this misperception by insisting that death is an unnatural event and failure to prevent it always constitutes therapeutic failure.

- End-of-life situations are a reality in intensive care. There is a population of patients who will die no matter what treatment is afforded them in an ICU. Sustaining these patients on life-supporting hardware results in pain, suffering, and discomfort, and the cost issue, if it exists, is not relevant. Technological life support for patients predicted to die does not equal comfort care, and comfort is always the most desirable therapeutic conclusion.

- Relatively few surrogates demand ineffective end-of-life care out of a desire to manipulate. Most surrogates who insist on medically inappropriate care do so because they have not been properly educated by physicians in charge. When physicians are universally placed in positions of medical directorship for intensive care medical services, their expertise in end-of-life care will facilitate achievement of patient and family educational goals and expectations.

Index

Copyedited and designed by
Katharine R. Wiencke